L

Live More Happy

Discover Yourself, Simplify Your Life and Set Yourself Up For Success

MAX MASON

MAX MASON

financial, medical or professional advice. The content within this book has been derived from various sources. Please consult a licensed professional before attempting any techniques outlined in this book.

By reading this document, the reader agrees that under no circumstances is the author responsible for any losses, direct or indirect, which are incurred as a result of the use of the information contained within this document, including, but not limited to, — errors, omissions, or inaccuracies.

ISBN: 9798585753787

Contents

LIVE MORE HAPPY

Introduction

I woke up on a lovely spring morning. But I was too busy to notice the crisp fresh air and the smell of apple trees blooming in my garden. I had a mission to accomplish. First, I had to drive my youngest son to school. I finally managed to wake him up, which is an accomplishment in itself, and we've rushed to the car to get going. I wanted to get to school as soon as possible, so I didn't even notice that I drove a bit more aggressively than usual, not thinking about the safety of my son or other commuters or even my own - I simply had to get there as quickly as possible without getting in trouble.

When I finally got there, I took him to class and rushed back to the car. I started feeling groggy, so I stopped at a coffee shop to grab a cup of coffee. I came back to my car, and I saw it was hit, but there were no other cars in sight. While I was waiting for the police to file the report, my friend called. He needed a lift, and of course I said yes. I'll be there soon, the police are finishing up filing the report as we speak.

I went to my friend's place, picked him up and started driving. He didn't even ask about the accident, but I didn't notice it back then and I didn't care. I had to drop him off at an underground parking lot, and on the last turn I clipped a column with the back driver side quarter panel of my car. Right on the other side of where my car was hit at a parking lot near the coffee shop just an hour ago. So I had nice symmetrical scrapes on both back quarter panels. Right at this moment I started realizing something, but I didn't know what it was.

I went back home, I came into my room and I froze. What do I have to do? Should I finish my paper? No, I still have time. Should I look for a body shop to fix my car? No, the insurance should cover that. Should I help my mother with the garden? I don't know, we've talked about it but I don't remember the details. My head started spinning. I felt so tired I fell on the couch and laid there for a couple of hours without even noticing.

When I finally found some strength to get up, I was angry at myself. I was breathing ragged breaths. I thought, how could I waste time when I have so much to do? And it came to me right there, right then. It was the first time in my life when I asked myself "why?". It wasn't the matter of "what". I knew what I had to do. I didn't know why I had to do it all.

It went further from there. I wondered who I actually was. My name is Max. Max is my name. I know that. But who am I, really? What do I stand for? Why am I doing what I'm doing? Back then, I realized I didn't even know myself. I realized I was the reason of my overwhelm.

I started realizing I should make myself my priority. I am a very kind person and I tried to help everyone whenever possible. But that day I realized people were using my kind nature to their advantage more often than I thought. In fact, I didn't even think anyone was using me. But then I remembered my friend didn't even care my car was hit, and he ran away when I clipped that column, because he was "busy" and had "urgent things to do". He didn't even call me back that day simply to ask how I was doing. And then I thought, why should I be his personal chauffeur? Why should I waste my time, waste gas, and risk my car getting hit when they don't even care about me? Why was I constantly helping everyone? Was I seeking validation? Is it simply because of my good nature? But why would I help someone when they don't appreciate it and don't even care about me? I felt frustrated, unsatisfied and unhappy even though I was busy all day trying to help everyone I could.

That's how I realized I needed to change my life. First, I had to discover myself. I couldn't even answer the question who I was, so that was the first logical step. Second thing I realized, I needed to make myself a priority and focus on self-care. Third, I needed to simplify my life by removing unnecessary commitments and toxic ungrateful people. I realized I couldn't help everyone. What's worse, many people were taking advantage of my kind nature. Fourth, I needed to find clarity on a lot of things. I was so overwhelmed, I didn't even know why I was doing what I was doing. And finally, I needed to set clear goals. I had to know what exactly I need to do and why I'm doing it. In short, I needed to focus on what was truly important to me and discard the rest.

In this book, you will find specific actionable techniques that helped a lot of people, including myself, to live more happy. Here's what you'll discover by finishing this book:

In Chapter 1, you'll learn how you can discover yourself and why it's important. In the frantic modern world, most of us walk around not really knowing who we truly are. When you discover yourself, you will discover your true values and goals. Discovering yourself allows you to avoid lots of frustration caused by putting time and effort into the wrong things. Once you discover yourself, you will gain more confidence in your abilities and will begin setting yourself up for success.

In Chapter 2, you'll discover how to make yourself your top priority and why self-care is important for your own well-being. Most of us have a mistaken belief that self-care is selfish. But you have to realize you have to take care of yourself before you can help anyone else. You can't perform at your best if you're tired, stressed, and frustrated. Maintaining a self-care habit is fundamental to creating a good life for yourself and the people who matter most to you.

In Chapter 3, you'll find out how you can simplify your life. Simplifying your life is important because everything in your life takes space, time and effort. Everything you do, everything you own and everyone you spend time with costs you something - time, energy, money. And when you have a lot of stuff, it costs you a lot. These days, our society reinforces the idea that the more we own, the happier we will become. In reality, most of us have more than we really need. Simplifying your life will allow you to find more time, space and energy. Living a simpler life allows you to enjoy the simplest pleasures.

In Chapter 4, you'll learn how to find clarity. Finding your purpose is one of the greatest feelings in life. And if you can actually pursue your purpose, you're on your way to living a fulfilling and joyful life. Finding your purpose starts with gaining clarity about who you are and what you want. Once you've established that, you can set goals that will allow you to pursue your purpose.

And finally, in Chapter 5, you'll discover how you can set yourself up for success by discovering your values, setting clear goals, and developing your strategy how to achieve them and stay focused along the way. Success is relative and can mean different things to different people. No matter how you define success, there are simple actions you can take to build on your natural preferences and strengths, guided by your true values and desires, and created by you in a way that would set you up for success.

By reading this book to the end, you'll discover how to live more happy by discovering yourself, making yourself your top priority and developing a self-care habit, simplifying your life and setting yourself up for success by setting clear goals and focusing on what's truly important to you.

Chapter 1: Discover yourself

Discovering your identity, discovering who you really are is the greatest and most important adventure of your life. However, many of us don't realize that and walk around not really knowing who we truly are. Even worse, some of us are always listening to an awful critical inner voice that gives us all the wrong ideas about who we are. We often think of self-understanding as something selfish and egoistic, and as a result, we fail to ask the most important question in life: "Who am I, really?".

Indeed, finding yourself may seem like a self-centered or even selfish goal. In reality, it is an unselfish process that is at the core of everything we do in life. In order to become the best version of yourself and succeed in various aspects of life, you first have to know who you really are, what your values are and what you have to offer to the people surrounding you and the world. Discovering yourself is a personal journey that everyone will benefit from taking. It involves breaking down and building up. Breaking down everything that doesn't serve you in your life and doesn't reflect who you truly are. And building up - recognizing who you want to be and fulfilling your destiny.

15

Discovering yourself is a matter of recognizing your personal power and being open to your experiences at the same time.

It may sound difficult, which is why many people tend to fear or avoid taking this fascinating journey. Yet, knowing yourself, knowing who you truly are, is the most important skill you can ever possess. When you discover yourself, you will discover your true values and goals. You will know what you need to do in order to achieve them. You will not have to seek validation or look for permission from others. Discovering yourself allows you to avoid lots of frustration caused by putting time and effort into the wrong things. Of course, life is naturally full of trial and error, however discovering yourself allows you to find the best areas for you to invest your time and effort in. Once you discover yourself, you will gain more confidence in your abilities and will begin setting yourself up for success.

Why it can be difficult to find yourself

There is a variety of reasons why it can be difficult to find yourself and know who you really are. Here are five most common reasons:

1. You were raised in a dysfunctional family that did not support individuality and had strict family roles.

2. You adopted limiting beliefs due to past negative experiences, and as a result, your self-confidence level is low.

3. You are influenced by various media, such as TV shows, YouTube videos, Instagram celebrities, movies and ads that make you think you have to be someone you are not.

4. You're surrounded by toxic people, which in turn reinforces your low self-confidence, inauthenticity and poor decision-making. This can lead to a vicious cycle of insecurity and confusion.

5. Your daily routine, habits and lifestyle prevent you from taking the time to disconnect, take a step back, and find who you really are.

Let's take a closer look at these points and explore them in more detail:

1. You were raised in a dysfunctional family

Most of your beliefs, behaviors, and values are formed during your childhood - your formative years. As a result, your childhood has a great impact on your adult life.

If you were raised in a dysfunctional family, it's highly likely you've developed low self-esteem and a weak sense of self. When a child has to be vigilant in order to protect itself against abuse or abandonment, they have no energy left to do the things children usually do: play, explore, and enjoy life. All their energy has to be invested externally in order to defend themselves. As a result, there is no inner energy left, and a child's identity becomes dependent on validation from the external world.

Dysfunctional families are characterized by having strict roles, where nobody is allowed to be an individual. Any deviation from what you are supposed to be is usually punished, and consequently, being an individual becomes associated with suffering.

Children in dysfunctional families are prevented from being themselves, they don't have authentic role models, and to make things worse, they are punished for trying to be themselves. It's not a surprise that deep down so many people are afraid of finding who they really are.

2. You have a low level of self-confidence

Low self-confidence level can be a result of being raised in a dysfunctional family or adopting limiting beliefs because of negative life experiences. Regardless, low self-confidence is often one of the reasons you struggle to find yourself.

Low self-confidence leads to a low sense of self-worth. Self-worth is essentially how worthy you believe you are. If you've adopted limiting beliefs such as "there's something wrong with you", "you don't deserve certain things in life", or "you're a bad person", it becomes incredibly difficult to discover who you truly are. Such beliefs can make you think you're not worthy of finding yourself.

In order to find yourself, you will have to purge yourself mentally and emotionally. We will discuss how to do it a bit later, but now let's move on to the next reason why you may be struggling to find yourself.

3. You're heavily influenced by the media

Nowadays, media dominates our lives. It is omnipresent. It's on the TV, radio, social media, it even surrounds you when you're walking on the street - you're being constantly bombarded by ads, billboards and screens.

One thing different media have in common is the message they send us. If you take a closer look, you'll see it's always about making you feel like you need more. More clothes, more shoes, more devices, slimmer body, whiter teeth - more, more, more.

On a deeper level, the message is that you're not good enough as you are. Companies, publishers and online personalities are all interested in making you unsatisfied with yourself in order to make you forget who you are and sell you products that supposedly will make you and your life better. They create certain images and make you chase them. It makes them a nice profit, but you lose yourself in that chase for the perfect image created by them.

Media is interested in making you feel insecure. They want to make you forget who you truly are and make you chase images created by them. It makes them powerful and important, but without your insecurity, they wouldn't have that.

4. You're surrounded by people who reinforce inauthenticity

There is a saying - good character is corrupted by bad company. We tend to attract those similar to us, and who feel the same about themselves that we feel about ourselves.

If you have low self-confidence, if you don't know who you are, you will attract people similar to yourself. It happens because ego needs validation, even if that validation is unhealthy and toxic.

Being around people who are confused about themselves can be comfortable, as it's usually non-confrontational. This is why we can feel intimidated when we're around a person who has a calm and grounded presence. We feel vulnerable and insecure because we haven't found that powerful presence within ourselves yet.

Your mental environment, the people that surround you and with whom you interact on a daily basis, can make it hard for you to burst out of that comfortable bubble and explore who you truly are. Many of us prefer to go with the flow and allow those surrounding us to dictate how we should live our lives. We can get used to it and find it comfortable, as living like this doesn't require a lot of effort. Moreover, we can be afraid that if we embark on the journey of discovering ourselves, we will lose our friendships, even though they can often be toxic and unhealthy.

5. Your daily routines, habits and lifestyle

All the previous points usually result in unhelpful habits and routines. Our lives can easily become cluttered by empty and meaningless commitments.

These choices can lead us into a sort of prison. They can make us feel stuck and trapped. They chip away at our self-confidence and reinforce inauthenticity. It can be very difficult to free yourself from them. But it is possible.

Let's explore how you can overcome all of these challenges and finally discover yourself, and know who you truly are.

How to find yourself

Life is too short to be someone you're not. Being who you truly are is a breathtaking experience. So many things in your life will start flowing beautifully once discover your true self.

All areas of your life will improve: your work and career, your relationships, your family life, your mental and emotional wellbeing, and most importantly, your relationship with yourself.

At this point, you're probably wondering how you can do that and finally discover who you really are. Here are eight steps you can take to find yourself:

1.   Make sense of your past
2.   Make time for solitude

3.   Purge yourself mentally and emotionally

4.   Determine what you really want in life

5.   Ask yourself self-discovery questions

6.   Embrace your right to be self-sovereign

7.   Remove people who reinforce inauthenticity from your life

8.   Silence your critical inner voice

This can be used as a step-by-step guide, however, you can attempt these steps individually. You have to remember some of them will work you, and some probably won't. You will have to experiment and find what works best for you. Don't be afraid of setbacks or failure, if you fall down, get back up and try again.

1. Make sense of your past

You have to know your own story and roots in order to discover who you are and why you act the way you do. You have to be brave and willing to explore your past, because this is an important step on the way to finding yourself and becoming who you want to be. It's not just the things that happened to us that make us who we are today, but rather the meaning we've made of those events. Negative experiences and unresolved traumas affect the way we act today. Research shows that life story coherence has a significant influence on our psychological well-being. Forming a coherent narrative of our lives gives us the ability to make more mindful and conscious decisions in our daily lives that reflect who we truly are.

We've talked about how most of our beliefs and behaviors are formed from an early age during our formative years. The atmosphere we grew up in has a profound effect on our adult lives. As children, we absorb the critical and hostile attitudes directed towards us. Such destructive attitudes become a part of our developing character and personality. As a result, we can develop a toxic alienated identity which opposes the manifestation of our true selves.

Negative life experiences, especially those in our childhood, establish how we define ourselves. They can influence our behavior in ways which we may not even be aware of. For instance, having strict parents can cause us to constantly be more guarded. As a result, in our adult lives we may always be feeling alarmed and resistant to trying new things because of fear of failure and being mocked. It's not hard to see how such behavior and attitude can distort our sense of identity and limit us in various aspects of life. To break this vicious cycle, it's necessary to determine and acknowledge what's causing it in the first place. We must be willing to establish the source of our limiting unhelpful tendencies.

Most of us try to cover up our negative past experiences, and as a result we can feel lost and like we don't really know who we are. We can even take actions and make decisions automatically without asking why. For example, you may lose your temper when interacting with your family or friends, it's quite a common occurrence. If you reflect on that incident later, you may find that such emotional outbursts have more to do with feelings you had as child towards someone who was unfair or hostile to you - your parents, your siblings, your teachers, your childhood friends or maybe even a stranger who scolded you. Our brain has many layers of meaning, and it's incredible how quickly old, and perhaps forgotten, memories and experiences can emerge in our behavior in the present. Such associations can make us act on autopilot without realizing or even asking why.

You can determine why you sometimes act on autopilot, and react poorly to seemingly innocent things, by reflecting on your past with a focused attention. In order to get off autopilot of ingrained behaviors and habitual responses, you should explore and label the emotions you're experiencing. Labeling is essentially naming and taming your emotional responses. You should not associate your emotions with yourself. They do not define you and they do not represent the truth. Instead of saying "I am angry", say "I feel angry". Instead of saying "I am sad", say "I feel sad". That is actually true, if you think about it. You should not let your emotions define you. Emotional responses can and should be controlled and used to your advantage.

By analyzing your experiences and emotions you can face your old memories and negative experiences and gain valuable insight into your behavior. You can consciously separate from the unhelpful or even harmful subconscious emotional responses. You can change and choose your responses and behavior to reflect your true identity, who you truly are.

2. Make time for solitude

Solitude is a powerful thing. It will not only help you reflect on your past in peace, but it's simply a relaxing experience.

In solitude, you can distance yourself from all the noise and fuss that clutters your mind and confuses you.

Solitude is simply being with yourself, with no distractions. No friends, no social media - nothing, only you.

It doesn't mean that you have to drop everything and become a hermit. Start by designating a couple of hours a week to being in solitude. Try your best to be alone. You can barricade yourself in a room or you can drive somewhere to be alone. Whatever you need to do to be alone - do it.

Of course, others can be confused or concerned why you need to be alone. Simply explain to them you need some time alone to rest and rejuvenate. Reasonable people will understand you, however you may have to set boundaries and find time to be alone in some cases.

3. Purge yourself mentally and emotionally

I found journaling is one of the most effective ways to purge yourself mentally and emotionally. I sometimes call it the vomit method. Why?

Because you have to vomit everything that you feel onto a page. Set no boundaries, just let in run free and don't censor yourself. You can get as explicit as you like.

Once you've done that, you can reflect on what you've written. Take a look at what themes are dominating and what emotions come through. You can use labeling here in a similar way as reflecting on your past. Determine what feelings are coming through and detach yourself from them.

Try to develop self-understanding. Don't be judgmental and don't worry if you're not completely sure of yourself. Just try your best to purge at this point.

4. Determine what you really want in life

We all have different desires, however our needs are essential to our survival and sanity. A good method to establish your core needs is to focus on the areas of life that lack the most and make you feel unhappy. If you feel miserable in some parts of your life, you can be sure a core need isn't being fulfilled.

Write down your core needs and think of all the ways how they are not being fulfilled. Determining your core needs is going back to basics. You have to remove of superficial desires and focus on what you truly need. This is what makes you, you.

Consider how rarely we make meaningful observations of what we like and dislike. We always complain, but in the end we still go along. Ask yourself: "What would create purpose for me?", "What would I like to be doing right now?".

We often forget what we really need in life. Not your parents, or your friends, your partner, your colleagues or society. You have to determine: what do you want?

You have to listen to your inner voice. Your life is yours to live. No one should tell you what you should and shouldn't want in life.

You can let your imagination run wild and think what you would do if there were no consequences. From there, you can make the appropriate compromises and determine your core needs.

We are naturally biased towards negativity. We tend to get overwhelmed by victimized thoughts and complain about our circumstances and surroundings instead of setting goals and finding solutions. Unfortunately, we tend to think a lot about what we don't want, instead of concentrating on what we do.

Discovering your needs and knowing what you want is essential to finding yourself. Recognizing your needs helps you discover who you really are and what's truly important to you. Yet, we tend to forget the most obvious things, and most of us rarely think about what we really want in life.

When you discover your core needs, you'll know how to direct your life and what goals you need to achieve in order to fulfill them. It is a vital step on the way to discovering who you truly are.

5. Ask yourself self-discovery questions

All your actions and all your thoughts are the result of questions you are asking yourself. For example, every day when you wake up you start asking yourself questions. Can I sleep five more minutes? Should I get up now? What should I eat for breakfast? What should I wear today? How is the traffic going to be today? What should I do later during the day?

You ask yourself these questions, and your mind finds an answer for each of them. These are all good questions, but they are not the most important ones. If you ask the right questions, your mind will look for the right answer. This is where asking yourself some self-discovery questions comes into play.

It's best to write down your answers so that you can come back to them later. Take something you can write or type on and let's get started. You don't have to answer all of the questions in a single sitting. You can always come back to them later.

Here are the questions you should ask yourself:

- If you were rich and had a lot of money, how would you spend your time and what would you do with your life?

- How does your perfect day look like?

- What are your hobbies, what do you love doing and what are you passionate about?

- What brings you joy in life?

- What things make you lose the sense of time and you can get totally consumed by?

- If you could live your life once more, what would you change and what would you do differently?

- What are the things that you regret that you did not do? Would you do it if you could turn back time?

- What do you like about yourself and what would you like to change?

- Do you see yourself as successful? Why and why not?

- Write down 101 goals that you want to accomplish before you die.

It may take a while to answer all these questions, however this is important because it will allow you to understand yourself better. Once you answer all these questions, leave them and come back to them the next morning after a good night's sleep. Review and read through your answers. Some of them may even surprise you. You will be amazed and feel great after doing this.

6. Embrace your right to be self-sovereign

Simply put, being self-sovereign means that you realize that only you are responsible for living your life, and no one else. You realize that only you decide what to do, and no one else. You realize that your life is created by you. Consequently, you have to remember that what works for others may not work for you.

Being self-sovereign means you have to assume the role of a king or a queen - a sovereign. Being a sovereign means you don't have to seek validation or approval from others, because you can find that acceptance within yourself.

It often happens that those of us who struggle to find themselves don't believe they can be self-sovereign. They believe that they need to adhere to society's norms and rules to be accepted.

Becoming self-sovereign is a rather simple mindset shift, but a very powerful one. It creates a massive change in your life. One of the best ways to becoming self-sovereign is determining who you are and who you aren't.

You can start by writing down your answers to the following questions:

- What is it that I like and dislike?
- What is my definition of success?
- How do I define happiness?
- What is beauty in my view?
- Who do I think I am and who others think I am?

If you have to think a lot before answering these questions, that's a good sign. It can take a lot of time and effort to find your true thoughts, feelings and beliefs and distinguish them from society's perceptions.

Another strategy you can use is differentiation. In simple terms, differentiation is a process of developing ourselves as independent individuals. We have to differentiate ourselves from destructive influences in order to discover ourselves and fulfill our unique destiny. Here are four essential steps to differentiation:

1. Remove negative personality traits adopted from your parents

2. Overcome defense mechanisms adopted from negative experiences during your childhood

3. Silence your critical inner voice

4. Develop your own values and beliefs, instead of accepting those you've grown up with

We've discussed how you can reflect on your negative past experiences in order to understand why you react to some things in a certain way and do things on autopilot. We'll discuss how you can silence your critical inner voice and discover your values later in the book.

7. Remove people who reinforce inauthenticity from your life

Considering you are the only one responsible for living your life, you have the right to find yourself, be yourself, and fulfill your unique destiny. You shouldn't let anyone drag you down. You should avoid poor habits and toxic relationships that can sabotage your efforts on the way to success.

Research suggests that you are the average of people you spend most time with. Consequently, you have to carefully consider who you spend your time with and what they bring to your life.

Make a list of all the people and commitments in your life at the moment. Analyze each entry in your list. Do they support you and improve you life or do they sabotage your effort to make positive changes?

Reworking your life fundamentally like this can be a scary task, but it's necessary if you want to make real changes. You have to find friends and commitments that will reinforce your right to find yourself and be self-sovereign.

8. Silence your critical inner voice

We all have negative thoughts from time to time, and they are often the product of our critical inner voice. Critical inner voice is a pattern of negative thoughts about ourselves, the others, our surroundings and circumstances, and the world in general.

Your critical inner voice has a massive impact on your life by undermining your self-esteem and self-confidence. It can destroy relationships, hinder your performance, and sabotage your progress on the way to success.

Your critical inner voice can manifest itself in all aspects of your life and in different forms. Some common negative thoughts are these: "You're stupid", "You're ugly", "You're weird". It can be about your career: "You'll never be successful", "Nobody appreciates your work", "You're useless". Many people experience negative thoughts about their relationships, such as these: "Your partner doesn't care about you" or "You're better off alone".

No matter what negative thoughts you might be experiencing, they all come from negative past experiences, that have internalized and formed the way you think about yourself. Here are the steps you can take to silence your critical inner voice:

Identify the critical inner voice

You can identify your critical inner voice by becoming aware of your inner self-talk about your environment and surroundings. For example, you can see your colleague in the morning and think about how they are always late and never do their job on time. Or you can be standing at a bus stop and thinking how your bus is late again and you hate public transport. This is your critical inner voice.

Once you have identified it, you can notice what comments and judgements it makes about yourself and your surroundings. Pay your attention to the thoughts that make you feel bad and bring your mood down. Try to determine what situations trigger the negative thoughts.

Establish where your critical inner voice comes from

Our critical inner voice is the result of past negative experiences, especially during childhood. Children absorb negative attitudes quickly and internalize them. You can notice that your critical inner voice uses the same phrases as you heard during your childhood. It can use the phrases you heard from your parents, your teachers, your friends and siblings.

Change how you react to your critical inner voice

Try not to fall down into a vicious cycle of negative thoughts that your critical inner voice tries to drag you into. Try not to engage in behavior that critical inner voice is telling you to.

Imagine you see someone at an event that you want to introduce yourself to. Your critical inner voice can say things like: "Why would they even talk to someone like you?". Notice that you've never even spoken to that person, so how could your inner voice already form an opinion about them?

Notice what your critical inner voice is telling you and challenge its comments and judgements. Remember that it can also encourage you to engage in destructive behavior. For instance, it can tell you to grab a few drinks before talking to the person you wanted to introduce yourself to. In that case, you can challenge this self-talk by telling yourself you have enough personality to interact with people without any drinks and you will feel better in the morning.

Use positive affirmations

You can use positive affirmations to reframe your negative self-talk. Write down some phrases and beliefs that your critical inner voice is telling you frequently. And then write down affirmations that are the opposite of those negative statements.

Dedicate some time throughout the day when you can repeat these affirmations to yourself for five minutes. It works best in the morning. You can stand in front of a mirror and repeat these affirmations. It may sound a little bit odd at first, but it works. You can meditate on these affirmations, repeat them when you're taking a shower or a bath or on your way to work. It will start feeling natural with time and practice, and you will notice your negative self-talk start diminishing.

Self-discovery is a fascinating journey, and it is the first step on the way to living more happy and focusing on what truly matters to you. Now let's move on to discovering how you can make yourself your top priority. Many of us have a mistaken belief that self-care is selfish, but it's simply not true. You have to take care of yourself before you can help others. With that being said, let's see how you can prioritize yourself and then how to set your priorities straight, so that you can focus on what's important to you.

Chapter 2: Make yourself your top priority

We should allow ourselves to be a bit more selfish. We should prioritize taking care of ourselves before taking care of others. We should make our own needs a priority.

We often fail to notice, but most of us are actually better at taking care of other people than taking care of ourselves. Imagine you were given a prescription. You will probably forget to take it from time to time. However, if prescription is given to your child or pet, you will always make sure they take it.

Most of us are bad at prioritizing our own needs over the needs of people around us. The majority of people work for other people, help their friends and family at the drop of a dime, and always reach out to help the people around us.

Let's stop for a moment and think, where does it leave you?

The answer is tired, stressed and frustrated. Because you didn't leave enough time for you in all your attempts to help everyone else.

This is why you should make yourself your number one priority. This is why you must become the most important person in your life. This is why it's always your first and everyone else second. Does that sound selfish? That's because it is. Being selfish is not a bad thing.

You have to take care of yourself before you can help everyone else. You can't perform at your best if you're tired, stressed, and frustrated. You can be of no service if you are exhausted from your constant attempts to help everyone. It doesn't matter how noble your cause may be, because if you're constantly drained, you can be of no use to anyone, even yourself.

On the contrary, if you take care of yourself and you have free time and energy, you can spare them to help others. Because in that case you have excess. You have taken care of yourself, which means now you have excess time and energy to help others.

You can help others when you're authentic and energetic. If you're stressed, tired and frustrated, it's highly likely you will only hurt people around you. You can make good decisions when you're well rested and full of energy. On the contrary, you will make bad decisions when you're exhausted, and despite your best attempts to help, you will only hurt yourself and people around you.

You should build everything on a foundation of self-love, from which everything else will flow. If you love yourself, you will make yourself your top priority in your life. If you love yourself, you will not put up with toxic people and destructive habits. If you love yourself, you will not subject yourself to unnecessary stress. Because you know that is what's best for you.

However, most of us don't know how to prioritize ourselves. We may be good at helping everyone around us, but we forgot how to take care of ourselves.

Why we fail to prioritize ourselves

Sooner or later we become stressed from running around taking care of everyone around us. The best thing we can do in this case is stop and think how we can take care of ourselves.

Sounds obvious, doesn't it? Nevertheless, the majority of people struggle with the idea of putting themselves first. It happens because most of us were taught to put others before themselves. We were taught that prioritizing your own needs is arrogant, selfish and is a bad thing.

This is the main reason why self-care is often overlooked, even though it is the essential practice for your own well-being.

Let's take a look at some misconceptions about self-care that might be holding you back from looking after the most important person in your life - you.

1. We think self-care means being selfish

Taking care of yourself is not selfish, it is your basic essential need, because it strengthens you and allows you to take better care of the people around you. If you are exhausted, you are of no use to anyone. Self-care is vital to reduce stress levels and maintain a healthy lifestyle. It allows you to improve your resilience so that you can better cope with challenges.

Remember how they tell you to put on your oxygen mask first on an airplane before you can help others? Self-care works with the same basic principle. You have to take care of yourself first before you can help others.

2. We confuse saving and caring

We often neglect self-care because we always try to save everyone else. However, you have to understand that this may not truly be in their best interests. We all have to learn our lessons in life, no matter how painful that may be. You shouldn't decide what's right for other people and stop trying to run others' lives.

You might think you're saving them from unpleasant experiences, but you have to remember you are denying them the opportunity to learn from mistakes and face their own challenges so that they can grow stronger.

It can be a hard truth to face, as you might think you are always being nice and caring. It can be even harder if it involves your family members or someone close to you. It's natural that you have an overwhelming desire to help, but what you need to realize is that they have to want to change. Nothing will change unless they realize they need to change and take action to make positive changes in their lives.

By saving someone every time you are enabling them to stay helpless and burn yourself out with stress. Of course, it doesn't mean you shouldn't help people. But you have to remember the difference between helping someone in need and taking it upon yourself to save somebody and make their life turn out the way you think it should.

3. We are used to relationships based on neediness, not love

Ironically, we often fall in love with the very idea of being in love. It happens because the media portrays love as something overly dramatic and needing to be with someone all the time.

In real life, not only is that impossible but also counterproductive. When we try to give someone all we have, we give too much, which leaves us totally drained. Instead of spending all the time thinking about your loved ones and forgetting yourself, you should focus on the most important person in the world - you. When you take care of yourself, you will be able to give your loved ones all the love and care they need, without expecting anything in return or feeling resentful.

Unfortunately, we often confuse love with dependence. In fact, you can only love in proportion to your capacity for independence. Taking care of yourself makes you more independent, because you will have less need of getting attention and more capable of connecting with others.

4. We don't realize our actions show others how to treat us

Your actions and attitude towards yourself teach other people how to treat you. Your actions are sending certain signals. If you are known as a person who always comes to help and will sacrifice yourself to help others - you will attract people who want to be saved. As a result, you will attract people who take advantage of your good nature.

At this point, it is necessary to question whether they took advantage of you, or you voluntarily gave it all to them. Maybe they pretended to be in need and took advantage of you. Maybe they really needed help, but then again, you can't save everyone. It can be hard to hear, but it's true. They played their part, but you can't change them. However, you can change yourself and your behavior.

You have to remember there is always a pay-off for us. Take a look and think whether you want to be a nice guy or a victim. Of course not, so start changing your behavior so that people wouldn't even think about taking advantage of your good nature.

5. We expect others to take care of us

When we take care of others, we may believe we are being altruistic and caring, but at the same time, do we expect something in return? You can give everything and be nice, but then feel resentful when you get nothing in return.

You probably know someone who always complains that people are ungrateful and they get nothing in return, even though they always help everyone. Maybe you experienced something like this. It's easy to complain about others and how ungrateful they are. But it's hard to realize and accept that you chose to give all your love and care to them and keep none for yourself, expecting they will reciprocate your generosity.

Of course, some people can take advantage of your good nature, but only if you let them. If you lie down to be walked on, you shouldn't be surprised if people treat you like a doormat. Only you can take care of yourself and no one else. Your self-care is your responsibility.

Why you need to prioritize yourself

Most of us were taught that taking care of others and being selfless is a good thing. But we have to remember that everything is good in moderation. Sometimes, we tend to take things to extreme. We push ourselves to the limit, we are trying to be productive and neglect our needs. Such sacrifices have a negative impact not only on your mental and physical well-being but also those who are important to you. Maintaining a self-care habit is fundamental to creating a good life for yourself and the people who matter most to you. Here are the reasons why self-care is essential for your well-being and those around you:

1. When you feel tired, you have nothing to give

When you are constantly running around trying to help everyone, you quickly lose your energy and desire. There is a difference between giving from a feeling you have something to offer, like helping a colleague at work or helping a stranger who is lost find their way, and making yourself do something because you should. The tasks remain the same, but your attitude changes.

If you take care of yourself and your needs, it is more likely that you will do your best to help people around you. On the contrary, when you do something because you should, you are not genuinely engaging in the process. It doesn't feel rewarding, and all you're trying to do is finish faster. This is why it's important to take care of yourself and your needs first.

2. Doing what you love empowers you

When you're happy and excited, you feel more energized and can offer more to the people around you. Doing what you love empowers you and brings a sense of joy and fulfillment. Just because it feels good, doesn't mean it's selfish or that it denies others. On the contrary, if you practice self-care and tend to your own needs, you change the way of how you relate to others. People around you get to experience the best version of yourself when you're fulfilled, happy and present.

3. We overwork ourselves to the point we lose our real selves

It's highly likely you know a person who goes above and beyond for their kids, their partner, or their job and career. They can literally follow their kids every minute of their day to cook for them, drive them to school and help them with their homework. They can do everything to impress their partner or their boss at work.

However, when we fall into this never-ending "do, do, do" cycle, we forget what makes all this hard work worth it to us. When we sacrifice ourselves like this, we lose ourselves. As a result, people around us can miss out on really knowing us.

4. We can drain others when we don't take care of our own needs

When you fail to take care of your needs, it can reflect on those around you. For example, when parents dedicate their entire lives to their kids, they later put a lot of pressure on them to fulfill their lives and desires. This is why adults should get their needs met by other adults.

It's much better for everyone when kids can witness their parents as fulfilled people. This way, parents can lead by example instead of making their kids fulfill their failed desires.

This is true in all kinds of relationships. If you neglect practicing self-care and taking care of your needs, you will have less energy, feel exhausted and complain about yourself and others, all of which is draining people around you.

5. We lose ourselves to our critical inner voice

We've discussed how your critical inner voice can drive you into a vicious cycle of negative thoughts. But there is more to it than that.

You can find yourself being preoccupied to be productive, and it may seem like a good thing. However, you have to take a look at what's pushing you. Do you do it because it makes you and people around you happy? Or is something else driving your desire to be helpful and productive?

Sometimes your critical inner voice can tell you that you have to meet certain criteria or achieve certain objectives to be worthy and accepted. It can reinforce the idea that anything you do for yourself is selfish, which is the main the reason many people neglect self-care. Your critical inner voice can be the catalyst to your unrealistic desire to be perfect and always put others first.

6. We neglect practicing self-compassion

You can become lost in all the things you think you should be doing for others. As a result, you can stop feeling for yourself. Research suggests that being kind to yourself and practicing self-compassion is one of the cornerstones of your well-being.

Having a kind attitude toward yourself gives you the ability to better learn from your mistakes and make real changes. Self-compassion allows you to accept your thoughts without becoming overwhelmed by them. You should stay attuned to yourself and avoid judging yourself too harshly. Practicing self-compassion makes you feel more comfortable being yourself, and as a result, that improves not only your own well-being, but also the well-being of people around you.

7. Our stress hurts us and people around us

It's no surprise that constantly running around trying to help everyone can make you stressed out quickly. Filling your life with responsibilities can lead to an unstoppable cycle where being stressed becomes normal.

Unfortunately, these days we are becoming reluctant to managing our stress levels. What's worse, we accept stress as something that proves our value and performance. Needless to say, stress is not a badge of honor. It can take a serious toll on your mental and physical health. These effects can catch up with you unexpectedly and prevent you from enjoying your life, negatively affect your relationships and lead to unnecessary conflicts and tension.

8. Neglecting self-care impairs your performance

There is a lot of research that proves that people who don't practice self-care have trouble with focusing on one thing and are easily distracted. It's unsurprising that their performance suffers dramatically as a result of not taking care of themselves.

If you don't take care of yourself, you will not be able to perform well. Taking care of yourself not only makes your life better but also allows you to show up for others energized and happy.

It's important to remember that being kind to yourself and practicing self-care is not selfish. It is what allows you to be the best version of yourself and perform at your best. You will be able to give your best to the world only when you've taken care of yourself and your needs first.

Effective ways to make yourself your top priority

Before we move on to discussing the ways to make yourself your top priority, let me tell you a short story. Years ago, I was at home relaxing after a day of hard work. I heard my phone ringing, I answered the call, and it was a friend of mine. He was in panic because he was driving along and his car died all of a sudden. We later found out there was an oil leak. He mentioned he had to top up oil from time to time, and that he was told there was an oil leak, but he never got to fixing it properly. So, one day he forgot to add oil, and his engine exploded because there was no oil left. And it all started with a small leak.

You're probably wondering what's the moral of this story? It's quite simple - your car will break down without regular maintenance. We depend on our cars for daily transportation needs, so it's natural we do our best to keep them well maintained. Yet, most of us forget to take care of ourselves. Neglecting self-care can lead to similar consequences as neglecting regular car maintenance. When you prioritize yourself, all the parts of your life will run smoothly and work better. But if you fail to take care of yourself, you can find yourself burned out physically and mentally rather quickly.

Self-care begins with self-awareness. You should notice when you become too tired, when you need a break and when you need something. After all, who can take better care of yourself than you? You need to make yourself your top priority in order to be able to perform your best. Here are effective ways that will help you prioritize yourself and your needs.

1. Realize self-care is essential to your well-being and is not selfish

Your physical and emotional energy reserves are not endless. There is a point of diminishing return when you expend more energy than you have in your reserve.

When you're overstressed, your coping mechanisms weaken. As a result, it creates a ripple effect further reducing your productivity and efficiency.

Being overstressed, over-scheduled and simply tired leaves no time and energy for the things you know would be good for you, but you have to push them on the back burner. The more things you push on the back burner, the more you lose yourself in the "do, do, do" mentality. You push your real self into a black hole when you leave no time for yourself and your own needs.

Taking care of your own physical and psychological needs is the best thing you can do not only for your own well-being, but for everyone around you too.

2. Make non-negotiable rules

Make a list of things that will make your life better and stick to it. You can add time slots where you allocate time for you. We've discussed determining your core needs as a part of discovering yourself. You should add habits and routines that help you fulfill your needs. Here are some great rituals you can add to your daily routine:

Make mornings your "me" time

Before you go anywhere or do anything, do things for you. It can be anything you find useful to fulfilling your core needs. You can meditate, do yoga, do some exercise, go for a walk, or read a book along with breakfast. Before you do anything for anyone else, do what is best for you first.

Eat a good diet

Unfortunately hectic modern lifestyle makes us eat junk food because we are often in a hurry. Some people even struggle to find time to eat and have to eat while working. If you are your number one priority, you have to eat good food. Eating junk food means that you are prioritizing other areas of your life over yourself.

Exercise daily

It may sound simple, but if you are your top priority, you have to exercise. If anything gets is the way of exercising, it means that it is more important for you than taking care of yourself. If you think you don't have time, that's because you don't create time. The better you take care of yourself, the better you will perform at work and in other areas of your life, and the more opportunities you will have to advance. You have to take care of yourself so that you can perform at your best.

Voice yourself

Not expressing what's on your mind is the same thing as lying, because you are not telling the truth. You may have your reasons for keeping silent. Sometimes you don't want to hurt other person or you may be afraid of their reaction. However, if you don't voice yourself, you keep the truth to yourself, never expressing it, and hurting yourself in an attempt to help others.

Be proactive

It is true that the early bird gets the worm in all aspects of our lives. Proactive people set the tone in business, relationships and other areas of life. You have the control if you know what you want. You will do what you can to prepare so that things don't catch you off guard. Proactivity means you won't have to be reactive to the plans of others. It means you can put your needs out there before anyone else sets the rules.

Stick to the rules you created and you will notice how you start prioritizing yourself each and every day. It may seem like a lot of work, but you have to do it all at once. Start small and gradually add more and more non-negotiable rules so that you can take better care of yourself.

3. Simplify your day

You should realistically assess your capabilities. Taking on more tasks than you can handle will only leave you frustrated. Don't plan on doing too many things on one day. It can get too hectic and all it takes is one thing not going according to plan.

Focus on what you need to do first. You can sort things by categories: work, friends, relationships, and don't forget to make time for yourself. Add only as many tasks as you think you can realistically handle, without having to stay up late only to wake up cranky the next morning. Sort and organize your plans for the day, and remove anything that's unnecessary. Do only what you consider to be a priority and leave the rest for another day.

4. Take a time out

It's good to be alone sometimes. We've already discussed how solitude is a relaxing experience and can help you clear your head and gain focus. It gives you time to be with yourself on your own. Being alone gives you an opportunity to take care of your needs in peace. You will be able to pursue your passion and feel more fulfilled. All areas of our life are time consuming. It's nice to take a break once in a while and take some time for yourself to explore your feelings and grow personally.

5. Find a hobby, do what makes you happy

Time is in short supply for most of us and it can feel like there isn't enough time in the day to do everything and find a healthy balance between work, play and family. But let's be honest, we find time for someone or something we deem important, it's just a matter of priorities.

Having a hobby is not just passing your time. It's the time when you are truly enjoying doing the things that you are passionate about. It brings out the best in you. It can be a truly therapeutic experience. Having a hobby allows you to reconnect with your inner child and bring it out. Unfortunately, many of us have lost touch with it in all the rush of our hectic lives. You should make time for things that are at the core of who you are and what you stand for. That way you can be your true self and be aligned with your passions and values.

6. Ask yourself what you really need in the moment

There is a misconception about self-care that it has to look a certain way. Depending on what's going in your life, your circumstances and your core needs, self-care can take many different forms. It can be anything that fulfills your core needs. It can be going for a walk. It can be sitting quietly on a couch with no devices and no distractions. It can be taking time out to do some self-reflection. It doesn't matter which specific routines you incorporate into your life. The main thing is that you are taking care of yourself. The result is what matters, how you get there is not important.

7. Take a snowball approach

One of the biggest reasons why people fail to take care of themselves is they think they don't have enough time. In fact, you can make time and it's not as hard as it might seem at first. Try the snowball method - start with one small action and build from there. Small actions have both immediate and long-lasting benefits, as they help you build useful habits. For instance, deep breathing even for a minute can help you become more relaxed and calm. You can start building from there. Go for a five-minute walk. Then work up to ten or fifteen and so on - whatever your schedule allows.

8. Make it a daily habit

Self-care should not be an escape from a long week at work or an exhausting month. This way you will be totally burned out and no vacations will help you get back on track. Self-care should be a daily habit. If you practice it regularly, you won't have to escape your life at all. Self-care consists of small actions and decisions we make on a daily basis. Like going for a walk, taking regular breaks, not staying up late and going to bed on time. All these small habits help us feel well, be present and show up for things that matter felling rested and energized.

9. Practice self-compassion

Let's say you planned to go for a walk or meditate, but for whatever reason that didn't happen. Instead of beating yourself up, you should have some self-compassion, forgive yourself and simply try again tomorrow. Don't be judgmental and don't indulge in guilt tripping. Having self-compassion creates a ripple effect of healthy habits and behaviors, such as exercising, eating a good diet, better stress management and healthy sleep patterns.

10. Practice saying no

Setting boundaries and learning to say no are essential to prioritizing yourself and your own needs. It's not as easy as it sounds, though. If it was easy, you would have started saying no a long time ago, right? Learning to say no can take time and practice. If you can't find courage to say no right away, you can start with "buying time" response. Instead of responding with a clear yes or no answer, tell people that you are busy and you will get back to them later. This will give you time to make a more detailed response in line with your own needs.

Always remember that you matter, your life matters, your needs and desires matter. When you take care of yourself, you are in a much better position to help others.

How to set your priorities straight

Now that you know how to make yourself your top priority, let's take a look at how to set your priorities straight so that they align with your long-term goals.

We try to complete all tasks each day because we feel that all items on our to-do lists are highly important. As a result, we become limited by time to complete all those tasks. If you ever found yourself in such a situation, then you probably don't have a clear list of priorities.

You have to set your priorities straight so that you can manage time effectively and know what you have to do to advance towards achieving your goals. Taking on too many tasks will stress you out eventually, and as a result, you won't advance towards your goals.

Your goals are essentially targets you want to meet in the future. Priorities are what allows you to focus on reaching that target. Once you set your priorities straight, you will be able to make changes and take the necessary decisions that are in line with your goals.

Everyone is different, of course, and everyone cares about different things. However, we all have some common threads that connect us all. Below you will find a list of priorities that are important for your own well-being as well as the well-being of those around you. Perhaps not all the priorities on this list will resonate with you, but you do not have to implement them all. Choose whichever fit your situation the best. Furthermore, if you're not clear on your priorities, this is a great list that will help you identify where you should focus your efforts and energy.

1. Your life missions

Your life mission is essentially what gives you meaning and happiness. It's what makes your life meaningful beyond being successful. Think about what you want from life. Determine your life mission and identify things you need to do to accomplish it.

Once you have determined your life missions, organize the tasks you need to do to achieve them. If something does not align with your life missions, consider eliminating it. Your life missions do not have to be something massive, epic and heroic. Maybe you've been overweight and want to lose weight. Go ahead, make it your life mission. It takes a lot of time and effort to reach that goal, and there is nothing wrong with making it your life mission. Or maybe you want to improve your public speaking skills. Make it your life mission and commit to practicing that. The bottom line is that all your tasks should be aligned with your personal and professional goals.

2. Physical health

Your health is highly important and should be on the top of your list of priorities. It affects all areas of your life: your comfort, your prosperity and your overall well-being and attitude. Bad health takes the joy and happiness out of your life and negatively affects your personal effectiveness and productivity. It's incredibly important to maintain your health in good condition.

It all may sound so obvious, yet most of us neglect their health in pursue of tasks that are not aligned with our goals and superficial pleasures. Here are the reasons why your health should be your main priority:

• Being healthy allows you to perform your best

- Your quality of sleep will improve

- You will be in a better mood when interacting with other people

- You will have more energy to accomplish your life missions

- You will feel more confident

There are simple things you can do to maintain your health. Eat good food and maintain a healthy diet. Remember to take regular breaks and develop an exercise routine. Go to bed at a reasonable time and don't skip sleep. Sticking to these simple things will greatly improve your health and well-being.

3. Spend time with your family

When you're going through tough times or simply having a bad day, your family is your first pillar of support. It's important to spend quality time with your family, as it improves your self-esteem, promotes positive habits, and allows you to create valuable memories.

Make spending time with your immediate family a priority and make that time count. Do some things that you enjoy together: go for a walk, exercise together, watch a movie together, cook together or simply have a meal together. Prioritize being together.

You can have a successful career and still spend quality time with your family. Try to avoid sacrificing your family while you pursue success at work or in business.

4. Healthy relationships

People are social creatures, and relationships play an important role in our lives. After your family, your friends and colleagues play significant roles in your life.

Prioritizing healthy relationships is like building pillars of support that will support you during difficult times. Healthy relationships reduce stress and help you cope with difficulties better. Studies suggest that people who maintain healthy relationships are less likely to experience psychological stress and their levels of stress hormone cortisol were considerably lower. It's not surprising at all, as we all know, social and emotional support that healthy relationships provide can help us handle stress better.

In addition to that, healthy relationships promote healthy habits. In healthy relationships your friends, colleagues, mentors and teachers have your best interests in mind. Try surrounding yourself with people that inspire you and avoid toxic relationships. We will talk about removing toxic people from your life in more detail in the next chapter.

5. Mental health

If you're always busy with work or studies, commitments, family and daily activities, you need to take pay attention to your mental health. You can do the following things to establish how you feel when you are busy and overworking, and keep your mental health in check:

Perform a mental audit

Take note and write down what you feel, think and say and whether it affects your mood in a positive or a negative manner.

Identify red flags

Red flags are signposts that indicate when you are experiencing a shift in your thoughts, feelings and habits. They can also serve as a warning when you are experiencing stress or burnout. It's important to establish what could be wrong, as it will allow you to develop strategies to resolve any issues you might be facing. The earlier you do it, the easier it will be to keep your mental health in check and get back on track.

Determine your trigger

If you notice that some tasks, events or habits, such as overworking or relationship issues, affect your well-being, try to practice self-care during such periods. Remember, self-care is not selfish and it will help you recover from stress so that you can perform at your best.

6. Finances

Let's be honest, money plays a significant role in our lives. Whether money can buy happiness is a debatable question, however, what is definitely true is that you have to earn at least above what you need to be happy. Life can become miserable is you're struggling to pay the bills or feed yourself. That's why it's important to prioritize your finances.

Figure out assets that generate income and liabilities that deplete it. Then reduce your liabilities and increase your assets. Try to save as much as possible instead of spending money on things that are not essential. You can invest your savings in a low-risk project that will generate some passive income. With that being said, avoid debt as much as possible and always save something for emergencies.

7. Self-improvement

Constant self-improvement is the key to success, and it's not as difficult as it may seem. There are simple yet effective ways to improve yourself. You can read self-development books, learn new skills or watch TED Talks or educational videos. It's always a good idea to learn something outside your field. Here are the steps you can take to make a self-improvement plan that works for you:

Establish your goals

Make a general list of your goals and then break up this general list into more specific items. This way you can set realistic achievable goals, such as earning a certificate, learning a new skill, or even losing weight. Yes, self-improvement does not have to be about learning something new, it can also be about improving your physical health. After all, it is exactly what it sounds like - working on yourself to improve.

Focus on your strengths

Determine your strengths and what you lack to achieve your specific goals. Then establish why you want to achieve them and how it will benefit you.

Visualize achieving your goals

Have a positive but realistic vision with as many details as possible. It will help keep you motivated on your way to achieving your goals.

Make a plan

Think how you can get there, what is required, and how you can do it. You may have to learn new skills or finish a course. You have to define actionable steps you need to take in order to reach your goals. Break them down into smaller milestones, as it will make you more motivated and you can reward yourself when you achieve those milestones.

To sum up, you will have to sit down and list everything that is important to you to establish your main priorities. If you feel burnt out and it takes a toll on your well-being, you need to prioritize your health. If you're struggling with your finances, you will have to address debt and control your spending. If you feel you're living an unfulfilling life, you'll need to establish your life mission and move forward to accomplishing it.

The next step is to make a plan. You can think what you can do to avoid burnout, how to address your debt and what actions you can take to accomplish your life mission. Then, set aside time for these tasks that will help you achieve your goals.

Now, let's see why our lives can get complicated and how you can simplify your life to free up some space and time for what truly matters to you.

Chapter 3: Simplify your life

A few years ago, I decided to simplify my life. The idea of simple living made me think what I actually need in life. The main thing I discovered was that having less stuff and fewer obligations allowed me to free up time for the most important things. It allowed me to find more time for the people I care about, things I love and opportunities I want to pursue.

While simple living has its benefits, it is not for everyone. However, you have to realize that simplifying your life doesn't have to look a certain way. It definitely doesn't mean becoming a hermit and living in a log cabin in the middle of a forest. You can simplify your life to whichever degree you desire and in ways that best suit your needs. It doesn't matter what your lifestyle is, where you live and what you do - you can take steps to simplify your life to the point where you feel satisfied.

Simplifying your life is important because everything in your life takes space, time and energy. Whether we are talking about physical space, mental space or time, you only have so much room. Everything you do, everything you own and everyone you spend time with costs you something - time, energy, money. And when you have a lot of stuff, it costs you a lot.

Simplifying your life will allow you to find more time, space and energy. You will feel more free and will be able to truly enjoy and appreciate everything.

Simple living meaning and definition varies from person to person, and you can pick and choose what you'd like to simplify. You don't have to go all in and strip everything to the bare bones. For me, simple life means leaving only the essential and removing everything else, eliminating chaos and spending time doing what's important to you.

It means removing all the unnecessary stuff and leaving only the things you value. It means getting rid of some things so that you can spend time with people you care about and do the things you enjoy.

Adding simplicity is not a simple process however. It is a journey rather than a destination. Our lives change, so we have to adjust to the changing circumstances sometimes.

So how does simplifying your life look? There two major steps to it:

- Identify what's important to you

- Eliminate everything else

It may sound simple but it can be difficult to apply to different areas of your life. You will discover what steps you can take to simplify your life a bit later in this chapter. Keep in mind not every tip will work for you, and you are free to choose what works best in your situation. But first, let's take a look at the reasons why life gets complicated, as it will help us understand which steps would be most effective in adding simplicity to our lives.

Entropy – the fundamental reason why life is complicated

Before we move on to the steps you can take to simplify your life, let's explore the fundamental reason why life is complicated and why it's important to simplify it.

According to Murphy's Law, anything that can go wrong, will go wrong. It may seem like a common adage people throw around in conversations, but it is related to one of the greatest forces in the universe.

Life in general has a tendency to get complicated, cause trouble and make things difficult. Problems seem to come out of nowhere, and we have to seek solutions which requires time, effort and a lot of energy. Life seemingly never works itself out. In fact, our lives are becoming more complicated and start to decline into disorder instead of remaining simple and organized.

Murphy's Law is related to a force that is fundamental to the way our world works and it affects every aspect of our lives and every objective we pursue. It is the force that drives many of the problems we have to face and leads to chaos. It affects everybody's life. It's called entropy.

What is entropy? Simply put, entropy is a measure of disorder or randomness.

Let's say you have a box of puzzle pieces. If you dump them on a table, theoretically, it is possible that the pieces will fall perfectly into place and create a completed puzzle. However, it never happens in practice because the odds are overwhelmingly against it. Every piece has to fall in just the right space to create a completed puzzle. There is only one state where every piece in order, yet there is an infinite number of states where they are in disorder. Statistically, it is highly unlikely to happen at random.

Entropy is a measure of disorder and there is always an overwhelming majority of disorderly outcomes.

In addition to that, entropy always increases over time. Things naturally lose order over time. When left on their own, structures, machines, devices and even our lives will always become less structured and more disorganized. Buildings will crumble, weeds will overtake gardens, cars will rust and people will gradually age. Even mountains erode and their peaks become more rounded. It is inevitable that things become less organized over time.

Nothing escapes entropy in the long run. Everything will eventually decay and disorder will always increase.

The good news is you can resist the pull of entropy. You can solve a puzzle. You can clear your garden of weeds. You can organize everything in your life.

However, since life naturally moves towards disorder, you will have to spend time and effort creating stability, sustainability and simplicity. Relationships require care and attention to be successful. Houses and cars need cleaning and maintenance. Things will decay if you don't take care of them.

Considering that disorder increases over time, and it can be counteracted by spending time and effort, we have to think about the core purposes of our lives. We only have that much time, energy and resources available to us, and we have to use them wisely, creating useful sustainable types of order that can resist entropy. Maintaining order in constantly increasing chaos is not easy. Simplifying your life is one of the hardest things, because everything is pulling you to be more and more complicated.

Entropy increases over time on its own. Maintaining order requires time, effort and energy. That's why you have to focus on what's truly important to you, and discard the rest.

Entropy dominates our daily lives and explains many mysteries. Think about a human body. It's a collection of atoms that could be arranged in an infinite number of ways, and most of them would not be able to function and lead to life. Simply speaking, the odds are against our very existence. We are a highly unlikely collection of atoms, yet here we are, and it's truly astonishing.

Entropy can also help explain why art is so aesthetically pleasing. Pieces of art created by artists are a form of order which the universe probably would never generate on its own. The number of beautiful combinations is extremely small compared to the number of total possible combinations. It is extremely rare in the grand scheme of things. Beauty is rare and is highly unlikely in our universe ruled by entropy.

Similarly, entropy can help explain why marriages fail and families fall apart. There are many reasons why marriages fail - incompatible personalities, financial stress, lack of trust, infidelity and so on. Deficiency in one of areas can destroy a family.

To maintain a happy family, you need a certain degree of success in each area. This is the reason why all happy families are alike. Disorder can take many forms, but order exists only in a few.

You have a specific set of skills, talents and interests that are unique to you. However, we live in a society that was not designed with your abilities in mind. Considering the nature of entropy, it is highly unlikely you grew up and currently live in an environment optimized for your talents. The probability that life will present you with a situation that is a perfect match to your skills is quite low. In fact, most of the situations you encounter will not cater to your talents.

Situations when an organism is not well-suited for conditions it is facing are called mismatch conditions in evolutionary biology. We use common phrases to describe mismatch conditions, such as "bringing a knife to a gunfight", or "like a fish out of water". When you are presented with mismatch conditions, it is more difficult to overcome obstacles and succeed.

It's highly likely you will be facing mismatch conditions throughout your life quite often. Life will not be optimal in most cases. Maybe you didn't grow up in the right environment for your interests. Maybe you were exposed to wrong subjects, sports, or hobbies. It's quite possible you were born in wrong time in history.

Despite that, you can design your desired lifestyle. After all, you create your own life and optimal lives are created, not found.

Entropy explains why Murphy's Law seems to manifest itself so often in life. There are a lot of things that can go wrong. Difficulties in life do not happen because some force is conspiring against you or some planets are misaligned. It is simply entropy at work.

Life has its problems and it's nobody's fault. It is simply a matter of probabilities. Disorder can take many forms, while order only exists in a few. Considering how odds are against our very own existence, it's remarkable not that life has its problems, but how we can solve them all.

Life is complicated because we are complicated

Sometimes being simple is the most complicated thing. Before I started simplifying my life, I remember it being excessively complicated.

I said yes just to satisfy others. I always showed up to help others, despite the fact that many people took advantage of my good nature, which I only realized later in life. But better late than never, right? I tried to control everything and rushed from one place to another, trying to do everything and help everyone. Such frantic lifestyle started driving me insane. I felt burned out and totally exhausted. When I reached this breaking point, I decided it was the time to start simplifying my life and focusing only on the things that are truly important to me.

When I realized how unnecessarily complicated I made my life, I started noticing how a lot of people live stressful lifestyles. Here are some of my observations on the reasons why life can get complicated, and the things you might want to avoid:

We try to do more than we can handle

Trying to do more than you can handle and over-committing is one of the biggest mistakes people make that complicates life. It may be tempting to fill every second of your schedule in an attempt to be super productive, but you have to remember you have a limited amount of energy available. Don't overwork yourself, leave space and don't forget you have to take regular breaks.

We try to control everything

When you try to control everything, you have to spend a lot of time and effort with doubtful results. Sometimes you just have to let go, relax and appreciate things as they are.

We constantly seek validation

You should create a life that feels great to you. You are responsible for living your life and no one else. Then why would you seek validation from others and let other decide how to live your life? Don't be afraid to create a life that's good for you and disregard what others might think, it doesn't matter at all.

We spend time with toxic people

Seeking validation often leads to spending time with toxic people. If you have to seek validation, it's highly likely you have a low level of self-esteem and self-confidence. As a result, you will attract toxic individuals with similar issues. Carefully consider with whom you are spending your time, as you are the average of people you spend most of your time with.

We worry about our problems

Worrying about problems does not help you solve them. You should not focus on your problems either, you should focus on finding solutions.

We are afraid of letting things go

To simplify your life, you will have to make changes. You will have to let go of some things in order to create space and time for what really matters to you. Don't be afraid to let things go. The old has to go to make space for the new.

We focus on what might be instead of being present in the moment

Worrying about what might be and wondering about what could have been takes your focus away from what is. It doesn't help you at all. You can't change the past, but you can change your future by taking steps in the present, no matter how small. Be present in the moment. Be here now. You can only shape your future by taking action now, in the present.

We avoid tough and necessary conversations

Problems can only be solved if they are identified first. By avoiding tough conversations, you are simply tucking away the problem. It highly likely it won't solve itself. It might feel good in the short-term, but in the long-term you are looking at a massive pile of unresolved problems.

We sometimes neglect our priorities

Your priorities won't get done by themselves. You have to make time for what truly matters to you. Time for your partner, for your kids, for your family, for learning, for exercise, for doing what you enjoy. You should focus on your priorities and push aside everything else in order to make time. By eliminating things that might sound exciting but don't have much significance, you can make time for what really matters to you.

We tend to procrastinate

We all know that feeling of a lingering task cluttering our minds. There are many reasons why we tend to procrastinate - lack of self-confidence, perfectionism, anxiety. If you find yourself procrastinating, you have to work on eliminating that habit. Remove all distractions, sit down and focus on the task. You can start small, it can even be five minutes at first. Try 15 minutes next. Then 30 minutes. This way you will build a useful habit and focusing on the task occupies your brain with solving a problem. Remember, the felling of getting something done is so much better that the feeling from sitting around thinking about doing it.

We ruminate over our old mistakes too much

We do a lot of things in life and it's natural we sometimes make mistakes. We have to learn from all our experiences, especially from negative ones, from our mistakes. All the experiences you've had made you into the person you are today. So don't be afraid to make mistakes. Learn from them, laugh at them, and move on. Don't waste your time ruminating over something you can't change.

We compare ourselves to others

All people are completely unique. You are a unique individual. You should follow your own path, live your own life, and fulfill your unique destiny. Don't compare yourself to anyone else. It serves no purpose, and you don't know all the circumstances at play.

There is no limit to how complicated life can get. One thing always leads to another. Life is complicated because we make it complicated. And our complications come from our way of thinking, our brain.

In the process of simplifying your life, the biggest obstacle you will have to overcome is your mind. If you can get over it, you can overcome anything.

Ways to simplify your life

Now that you know why our lives can get overly complicated and why it's important to simplify them, let's take a look at the concrete steps you can take to simplify your life. Remember, there is no perfect formula of how to simplify your life. You have to take your own core needs, goals, and lifestyle into account. You can pick and choose what methods work best for you. With that being said, here are the steps you can take to simplify your life.

1. Declutter your house

Your physical environment plays a big role in how you feel. Having too many things wastes your time and resources. It makes you waste time by looking for misplaced items or getting overwhelmed each time you open your closet. A clean, organized space makes you more productive and energetic than when you're living among scattered piles of random stuff.

All your possessions cost you something - time, energy, money. And when you have a lot of stuff - it costs you a lot. This is why it's important to identify the most important and essential items and discard the rest. You'll feel lighter when you have less stuff to worry about. You will also have more time, money and energy for the things that are important to you. Start decluttering gradually, one room at a time. You'll soon notice how much easier it is to live when you rid of the things you don't need.

Most of us have more than we really need. Despite that, sales and the wow effect from seeing a gimmicky item make us add more to our collection. Our society is built on a belief that possessions will make you happy and impress people around you. This focus on consumerism and materialism makes your home and your mind cluttered. Take a look at your closet, for example. It's highly likely there will be things you've already forgotten about and haven't worn in a thousand years. Or even never worn since you bought them.

Take some time out to declutter. Go through your all of your possessions. Go through your house room by room. Consider donating some items if you can. Sell whatever is appropriate and throw away the rest. Some people have so many possessions that they forget they even have some items. Don't hold on to things that are broken and you're hoping to fix them someday. Or the things you haven't used in a while and keeping them just in case. Determine the things that are truly valuable and let go of the rest.

2. Remove toxic people

Negative people can take up a lot of space in your life and drain a lot of energy from you. Many of us probably have a friend who constantly finds themselves in trouble, or a cousin who always complains about how unfair the world is. Of course, you shouldn't cut people out of your life just because they are going through tough times. However, setting boundaries is important.

Even if you don't spend much time together, it still takes quite a bit of time and energy to meet them and then calm down after a visit. In some cases, the best thing you can do for yourself and someone else is to say no or cut ties altogether. Removing toxic people from your life makes space for those who are most important to you.

Relationships are complex and often require a lot of time and energy to make them work. When everyone is investing time and effort into a relationship, it's often worth the trouble. But if someone is draining your energy and only adds negativity to your life, you need to evaluate whether you want to spend time with them at all.

It can be difficult to remove people from your life. After all, we are creatures of habit. However, removing toxic people from your life is the kindest thing you can do to yourself and to them. It doesn't matter who they are. Whether it's friends, coworkers, your partner or family, a toxic relationship will only leave you damaged and drained. If you don't want to cut them out completely, try making a no-contact break first. If they don't respect it, then you know they don't have your best interests in mind. Do what you need to do. Cut the toxic people out of your life.

We tend to have more things and people around us than we really need. Removing toxic people and unnecessary things from your life will help you become more organized and efficient.

3. Review your time commitments

In addition to removing unnecessary things and toxic people from your life, you can also consider reducing the number of commitments. If you're struggling with running a carpool or having too many meetings, learn to say no. It's great to give back and spend time with your friends, but it's also important to have healthy boundaries, so that you can focus on the things that are truly important to you.

Many of us fill our days with commitments from beginning to end: work, business, career, home, family, kids, events, hobbies and much more. You should consider releasing yourself from commitments that are not in line with your core needs and values.

Our world moves at a breathtaking pace. Technology and communication develop faster and faster. We're getting overloaded with information and social media is ingraining itself into our lives every day. Expectations and demands continue to grow, but the number of hours in a day doesn't. Our lives get busier and busier every day.

Living a busy life will not benefit you in the long-term. Sometimes we are so busy we keep switching from one thing to another, failing to notice how overwhelmed our lives have become. This is unhealthy to say the least, and unfortunately we often don't recognize how busy and over-committed life is harming us. What's worse, is that we fail to identify hidden lies that keep us busy and overwhelmed. Here are nine hidden lies you should be aware of before reviewing your commitments.

Accolades bring fulfillment

We often think that the busier we are, the more we can accomplish and the more respect we will earn. And the more accolades and respect we earn, the better we can prove our worth to others. This is not true. If you're seeking validation and trying to find fulfillment in someone else's opinion of you, you will never find it. You will always have to search and work for more.

Money brings happiness

Don't get me wrong, money is important and everyone needs to provide for their own needs and the needs of their family. But it's foolish to think that money is the quickest way to better living. We often get caught up in trying to earn more money. You should control your finances and make money work for you. You should address your debt if you have any. But it's unwise to overwork yourself and undermine your health and well-being just to make more money. People are often trying to earn enough to buy things they are too busy to enjoy.

I don't have a choice

Many of us tend to seek validation from other people. As a result, we tend to live busy lives just because of the expectations and demands of others. In such cases, you have to remember you always have a choice. Of course, there are times when life will require more of you. But most of the time, we live overly busy lives simply to fulfill others' expectations. Consider who is really making decisions in your life and how you can regain control.

Being more busy means being more productive

It may be true for a short while, but people simply cannot work relentlessly for an extended period of time without rest. Rest is essential for productivity and finding a nice balance between being productive and having some rest is important. Otherwise, a constantly busy lifestyle will decrease your productivity and can even undermine your health and well-being. Don't forget to take regular breaks and have a good rest every once in a while.

Hold your pride

In simple terms, pride is holding an excessively high opinion of oneself or their importance. Pride can lead to overwhelmed life because of the foolish thinking along the lines of "I am needed" or "Nobody can do what I do". Pride negatively affects all areas of our lives: work, business, family, relationships and more. It leads to an unnecessarily busy life, and in the end, a fall. Focus on doing what's truly important to you, and not what your pride or ego tells you to.

Everything is important

In the modern world everything seems urgent, important and beneficial to your life. As we're getting overloaded with information, our brain starts failing to process, sort, and filter all that information. You have to realize you can't accomplish everything, and not everything is important. In fact, there are very few things that are truly important.

I need to be busy to keep up with everyone else

Sometimes it may seem that the only way to get ahead is to outwork everyone else. Even if everyone appears to be busy at all times, it doesn't mean they busy doing the important things. And it certainly doesn't mean they find joy and fulfillment in their pursuits.

Busy makes me look more important

Being busy in itself is not an achievement or a badge of honor. In fact, being busy doing things that don't matter is detrimental to your success and well-being. You don't need to be busy just for the sake of it. You need to focus on doing the things that will assist you in reaching your goals.

Quietness is laziness

On the other hand, people tend to think that quietness equals laziness. We're so used to the fact that something is constantly happening around us that we confuse quietness with procrastination or laziness. Quietness is not laziness. It's hard to achieve, and it's worth the effort. Spending some time alone in quietness is truly a therapeutic experience.

We believe many hidden lies that displace the things in life that matter most. Instead of enjoying a calm, intentional life, we rush from one needless thing to another. Review your commitments and focus on what's truly important to you.

4. Get rid of bad mental habits

Bad mental habits can have an enormous negative effect on your mental health. Dwelling on the past and feeling sorry for yourself are the most common examples of such habits.

We've already discussed how you can silence your critical inner voice, which is usually the reason for negative self-talk and bad mental habits. Clear the mental clutter and eliminate unnecessary negative self-talk. This will allow you to make space for healthy mental habits, such as self-compassion, positive realistic self-talk and gratitude.

If you find yourself engaging in negative self-talk, notice what your critical inner voice is telling and challenge its comments and judgements. Take a deep breath, remind yourself that negative self-talk is not helpful, and switch it to positive realistic inner dialogue.

5. Don't waste time on being negative

Unpleasant things can happen to all of us and turn the day from good to bad. Maybe you got splashed by a passing car, your boss scolded you in front of your colleagues or you missed a bus.

It's natural that we have a negative reaction to such things, but it's how you deal with these situations that can have a massive impact on your life. If you spend the rest of the day thinking about how bad those things were, you are simply wasting your time. Yes, it's really that simple. You can't go back and fix it, you just have to deal with the consequences.

The immediate negative reaction is natural, and it's totally fine. However, dwelling on those negative experiences is what really destroys your productivity and personal effectiveness. Instead of ruminating or feeling regret, you should just let it go and be more productive, so that you can use this time for things that matter to you. Moving past negative experiences can be difficult, but you have to find ways to focus your energy on moving forward.

Just think how much time you wasted by dwelling on past negative experiences and thinking about what could have been. Staying positive and finding ways to move forward can be difficult, but it's a very important way to simplify your life.

6. Unplug from technology and social media

These days it's hard to imagine living without our devices, even though just a decade ago none of this even existed. We used to interact with people and maintain eye contact to get things done. We used to read books, watch movies, and listen to music without getting distracted by a phone. We wrote letters and actually thought how we could best convey our feelings. Now, we just shoot text messages without even thinking about it.

I'm not saying you should get off the grid entirely - this is not realistic and often not necessary. However, you can make an effort to unplug from technology when it's not needed. Leave your phone in your pocket or purse when you're having dinner, for example. Try playing a board game instead of watching TV. Meet and talk to people in real life more often. Reconnect with yourself and others. Be present in the moment without being distracted by your phone.

Another aspect of unplugging from technology is social media. Think how many times you picked up your phone just to scroll through the same feeds for the thousandth time? We often do it on autopilot because it's so ingrained in our culture at this point. And it's quite sad, to be honest.

One of the common reasons that self-care gets neglected is that people think they don't have enough time. Yet, they find time to sit down and stare into their phone. You will be amazed by how much time you can gain if you simply put down your phone. In addition to that, try deactivating social media. It doesn't have to be permanent. Try doing it for a couple of days at first. While you'll get an uncomfortable feeling of not being connected, you'll find a lot of time for things that really matter. You will stop wasting your time on scrolling through the same feeds for no reason, and if somebody needs to get in touch, they can simply call or text you. Try putting your phone down and getting off social media, and see how much time you'll gain for the things that truly matter to you.

7. Create a morning ritual

We've talked about how you should make morning your "me" time. You can take it a step further and create a morning ritual. Instead of hitting that snooze button a few times, you can create a ritual that gets you to a more positive start in the mornings.

Prepare the night before: pack your bag, lay out your clothes and go to bed at a reasonable time. You can try setting the alarm half an hour earlier so that you can do something that will make you feel great. It can be going for a walk, doing some yoga, or simply drinking a cup of hot beverage, looking out the window and self-reflecting. Create a morning ritual, make it a habit, and you will reap the benefits throughout the day.

8. Start meal planning

Most of us know that sinking feeling when you're not sure what to eat. You have to think whether whatever you have in the fridge and pantry is enough to cook a meal, or just end up hitting a drive-thru or ordering takeout.

While meal planning may seem like a chore, it will save you a lot of time and money in the long-term perspective. Make a list of things that are easy to cook and are tasty to eat and start planning your shopping. You can shop on Sunday for the week ahead and then assign meals for every day. Stick with your meal plan and you will soon notice how much easier it is and how much time you're saving.

9. Take control of your finances

If you're not taking control of your finances, money will take up a lot of space in your life, and it doesn't matter how much money you have.

You need to take charge of your money. Create a budget and establish clear goals. It will help you make financial decisions much simpler.

Once you take control of your money, you will spend less time and energy thinking about it, and will make it work for you.

Another important aspect of taking charge of your money is addressing debt. It doesn't matter whether it's a credit card balance, a car loan or student debt. These days most people owe some kind of debt. Many try not to think about it and bury their heads in the sand, unaware of how much they really owe and when they will be able to pay it off. Obviously, such behavior is not helpful and it won't make debt disappear.

Get up close and personal with your debt. Establish how much you owe, learn about the interest rates and see if there are any options for lowering them. Take a look at your credit report and resolve any problems you find. Get in touch with your debtors and find out if it's possible to get your debt paid off faster. Face your financial problems head on and never ignore them. It will feel great once you reach financial freedom.

10. Gain control of your time

Time is the most valuable resource you have. You can never gain more time. Despite that, we waste it so easily dwelling on the past, complaining, mindlessly scrolling through social media, or waiting for things to happen.

Don't just go along through life being busy and passing time. Stop doing things that are wasting your time. Use your spare time to do things that matter to you.

But don't lose yourself in the "do, do, do" mentality. Leave some time for just being. You need some time off to clear your mind. Go for a walk, play with the kids, spend some time alone and do some self-reflection.

Be in the moment and use your time to do things that truly matter to you.

11. Spend some time in peace

Speaking of taking control of your time, we live in a constantly moving and changing world. We live in a fast paced, noisy environment. Think for a moment, when was the last time you sat down in silence without any distractions? For most of us, it's an incredibly rare occurrence.

Spending some time alone in silence can help you do some self-reflection, which in turn will help you relax and clear your mind.

For most of us, it can be difficult to find time and place where we could spend some time alone in silence. You can start small: turn off the radio while driving, stop constantly checking your phone and scrolling through social media, turn off the TV. You can go for a walk by yourself or you can drive somewhere if you'd like. You can even simply drive around with no destination late at night or early in the morning when there is little to no traffic, it can be a therapeutic experience.

Spending some time in peace will allow you to clear out the distractions and focus on what's important to you.

12. Start small and keep subtracting step by step

Life can get complicated and simplifying it can feel like an overwhelming task which is the opposite of what simplifying your life is about. Remember, you don't have to change everything and you don't have to do it all at once.

You don't have to go through all these steps. You can pick and choose whatever works best in your situation. Start removing one thing from your life every day. Get rid of some clutter, cut out toxic people, spend some time alone and clear your mind.

These days, our society reinforces the idea that the more we own, the happier we will become. In reality, most of us have more than we really need. Everything you own costs you something. Consequently, the less you own, the less time and energy you will have to spend on things you don't really need. Living a simpler life allows you to enjoy the simplest pleasures.

Now that you know how you can simplify your life to create more time and space for what's important to you, let's discuss how you can gain clarity. We often find ourselves confused in the fast-paced, frantic modern world. Gaining clarity will help you to discover your purpose and your passions, and find out what exactly is important to you and how you can achieve it.

Chapter 4: Find clarity

Finding your purpose is one of the greatest feelings in life. And if you can actually pursue your purpose, you're on your way to living a fulfilling and joyful life. We all have a unique purpose. The key to living a fulfilling life is finding your purpose and using it as a guide to move towards your passions and dreams.

Believe it or not, we all know our purpose, it's just buried deep inside of us. Our environment, people that surround us, various events, our way of upbringing and our inner self-talk can push our purpose so deep down that we may even think it doesn't exist. But everyone can find their purpose. It may take some time and quite a bit of effort, but you are capable of finding your purpose.

Moreover, we can have more than one purpose. And our purposes can change as our lives go on. It may sound a bit overwhelming, but let's focus on finding your current purpose for now.

Finding your purpose starts with gaining clarity about who you are and what you want. Once you've established that, you can set goals that will allow you to pursue your purpose. Unfortunately, with the hectic modern lifestyle, most of us don't even think about who we are and what our purpose is.

Although it may sound fairly simple, in reality finding your purpose takes a lot of self-reflection and constant personal growth. We may often fantasize about achieving their goals and dreams, but never take action to make that a reality. However, many people don't even know what they want and what their dreams are. And it's quite sad, to be honest.

Lacking clarity makes you feel stuck. It's possible you're feeling stuck right now. Unfortunately, confusion, distraction and disorganization have become a part of our lives. Let's take a closer look at what it all means:

- Confusion happens when you don't have clear priorities, and as a result you're unsure what to do next.

- Distraction has become normal in the modern world. It's a hundred small things that make it hard for you to focus and pull your attention away from what's important.

- Disorganization is the lack of orderly thinking that leads to reduced productivity.

The good news is, it all can be solved by gaining clarity, learning to maintain focus and simplifying your life and removing the unnecessary clutter.

- Confusion is solved by gaining clarity and setting your priorities straight.

- Distraction is solved by learning how to maintain your focus.

- Disorganization is solved by simplifying your life, eliminating the unnecessary and focusing on what's important to you.

You already know how to set your priorities straight and simplify your life. You'll discover how to set your goals and maintain focus in the next chapter. But first, let's find out how you can gain clarity and why it's important.

Confusion is the product of being lost in your thoughts. These days we experience so much confusion that we think it's becoming the norm to be confused in our complex modern world. In reality, you have more clarity than you might think. You have to get out of your head and start digging to gain clarity. It will help you find your purpose, set actionable goals and pursue them.

What is clarity?

If you search for the definition of "clarity", you'll get a lot of different answers. Clarity can be defined as the quality or state of being clear or as freedom from indistinctness or ambiguity. But these definitions are far too complicated. After all, clarity is all about clearing confusion, and these complex definitions only bring more confusion.

So, let's see how we can simplify the definition of clarity. Speaking of simplifying, clarity and simplifying go hand in hand. One of the definitions of clarity that caught my eye was the quality or condition of being clear or easy to understand. That's a better definition for a word that should be so simple. However, I think we can do better than that.

The simplest definition I came across was that clarity means clearness. This is it. It makes sense and is easy to understand. Clarity is clearness. That's it.

What is mental clarity?

Have you ever experienced that you are living in a thick fog, not knowing where you're going? Did you ever get a felling that you can't concentrate, your mind was constantly racing, and it was so hard to make decisions? All these things are the opposite of having mental clarity.

On the contrary, when this fog lifts, your mind becomes calm, and you feel empowered to make decisions. That's mental clarity. It may sound simple, yet with so many distractions and stress it can be hard to get there. Let's discover how you can gain clarity, but first, let's see why we can get confused in the first place and how we can overcome it.

Why we become confused

Being confused is not the greatest feeling, and most people don't like it. It's like being in a thick fog, not knowing where you're going. You don't know where to go, what to do, and you feel overwhelmed by problems with no solutions in sight. Not knowing what to do next is one of the most unpleasant feelings.

But what is confusion, and where does it come from? Confusion comes from your mind. It comes from thinking. When you feel confused about what choices to make, it may seem logical to try and think your way out of it. But this is a mistake, and here's why.

There is a situation playing out on one level. Then layered on top are your thoughts about that situation. We feel confused when we can't make sense of what's happening. When you're confused, it means you've probably slipped into overthinking, and trying to think your way out of it won't work. Feeling confused is actually a signal to stop thinking for a moment.

Because confusion is the product of thinking, thinking will not solve it. Confusion can clear itself eventually, but you spend more time being confused if you indulge in habits and behaviors that feed it. Things like dwelling, ruminating, and over-analyzing only promote confusion.

Trying to think your way out of confusion is tempting and may seem like a logical thing to do. It makes your brain occupied and makes you think that you are actively seeking a solution to the problem. But it only seems so because you are already confused. When you are in a state of confusion, all the options you think are available to you will only lead to more confusion.

You can find a solution by analyzing your way to it, but you cannot gain clarity by analyzing. A solution born of confusion is very different from a solution born of clarity.

Solutions born from confusion are usually short-term fixes, they don't resolve the problem fundamentally. Solutions born from clarity tend to be fundamental and innovative. They take you forward, while solutions born from confusion make you come back to the same old problems over and over again. If you want real lasting solutions, you have to gain clarity first.

It may seem that confusion just happens to us. We think it's real, like all the objects that surround you. In reality, confusion is only an emotion created by our thoughts. It's not a state of being. Confusion is just an emotional response to our unwillingness to take responsibility for making decisions. We are afraid to take responsibility because we become terrified thinking about what if it's a wrong choice.

We also stay confused because we let the future circumstances affect and create our feelings. We think that circumstances created by our choices will affect our feelings. As a result, we believe we can't manage our minds in the future and accept the consequences of our choices. Confusion is usually a sign of an unmanaged mind.

First, it shows that you are not managing your mind because you accept "I don't know" or "I am confused" as an answer. As a result, you believe you can't overcome your confusion and that a solution will magically appear our of nowhere.

Second, you think that you will not be able to manage your mind in the future as well. Instead of deciding how to think and feel, regardless of the circumstances or results created as a result of your choice, you leave yourself at the mercy of your unmanaged mind in the future.

You can stop being confused, and it's really simple. All you have to do is to decide.

First, don't take "I don't know" for an answer from yourself. Stop it. This way you train your brain to turn off when it's faced with a problem and you need to make decisions. Your brain will always choose to just say "I don't know" if you keep doing it.

Second, eliminate the belief that you are confused. Confusion is an emotional response. You don't feel confused because you have all the different options and you have a decision to make. You feel confusion as an emotion because you're actually making yourself believe you're confused when you say "I am confused" in your inner dialogue.

In order to eliminate confusion, you have to understand and eliminate the source of confusion. There are two types of confusion and two different thoughts underlying them.

The first is confusion about what others are doing, saying or thinking.

The source of this sort of confusion is the underlying thought that you need to understand what others are doing, saying or thinking. You can decide what to think and feel for yourself, regardless of what others might be doing, saying or thinking. You don't even need to know what they are doing, saying or thinking. All you need to know is what you want to think, how you want to feel, what actions you want to take and what results you want to achieve. If you know that, you can come up with concrete steps to achieve all of that.

The other type of confusion is the thought that you can make a right or wrong decision. There is no such thing as a right or wrong decision. How do you know if it's right or wrong? How do you determine that? Let's imagine you find yourself in new circumstances as a result of your decision. Your brain looks at the results and says "well, that was a mistake". You have to realize it's just a thought. Our thoughts often do not represent objective reality. Your brain analyzes everything it sees and judges whether it's right or wrong. It's just a thought and nothing more.

Whatever thoughts you might have, you can manage them. That's what it all about.

Confusion is the product of our mistaken belief that one decision is right and the other is wrong, and your success and happiness depend on choosing the right one. But it's not true. Your success and happiness depend on your thoughts. And when you realize you can choose how you want to think and feel, there's no reason to fear the future.

Why clarity is important

Gaining clarity sounds great and it may seem fairly obvious why it's important, but there's more to it than finding your purpose. Here are reasons why gaining clarity is important:

- Having clarity helps overcome doubt and improves your level of self-confidence

- It helps you avoid or reduce frustration, because when you have clarity - you have less confusion

- It allows you to determine your strengths and weaknesses through self-reflection, which in turn helps you start and maintain the process of constant self-improvement

- You need clarity to set goals, lay out a plan and take action, clarity is essential to moving forward in life

- With clarity you can make better decisions that are aligned with your core values and make them faster

- Clarity helps you avoid getting stuck and helps you keep moving forward when you feel stuck

- Having clarity lets you feel more energized and focused in your daily life

You've probably heard about how important it is to have a positive mindset, however I think the key to success is a clear mindset. When we experience confusion, a lot of our brain space gets occupied by uncertainty. Mental clarity helps you overcome confusion and free up your mind. Gaining mental clarity is important for the following reasons:

1. Mental clarity helps you focus and find direction

We all experienced confusion and we all know how lost you can feel and how hard it can be to find direction and make progress. When you gain clarity about your goals and priorities, it will be much easier to lay out plans on how to achieve them and take action.

2. Mental clarity makes it easier to take action

When you have a clear reason why you have to do something, it's so much easier to take action and get things done. Many of us have started something only to give up halfway through. It usually happens when you're not clear why you were doing it in the first place.

3. Mental clarity makes it easier to prioritize

When you're in the fog of confusion and are overwhelmed by indecision, it becomes incredibly hard to make choices that will allow you to move forward. Having mental clarity helps you organize overwhelming possibilities and determine how you can resolve the necessary tasks. It helps you make decisions instead of overthinking and digging yourself deeper into confusion.

4. Mental clarity helps you overcome doubt

It's easy to start doubting when you're feeling distracted and lacking focus. Mental clarity allows you to be honest with yourself and see yourself honestly and without judgement. Mental clarity helps you stay focused regardless of what others might think about you. With mental clarity, you won't even entertain these thoughts.

5. Clarity allows you to feel content

Mental clarity allows you to see and appreciate things as they are, instead of wondering whether you are doing good enough or if you are good enough. It provides awareness which allows you to enjoy and appreciate little things that are often left unnoticed and feel more content with whatever is going on around you.

With that being said, here are five signs that you lack mental clarity:

1. You always question yourself and your actions
2. You constantly have to ask others for advice
3. You're unsure about your priorities and say yes to everything
4. You're often overwhelmed with ideas and possibilities and don't know what to prioritize first
5. You abandon different projects halfway through and struggle to bring them to completion

In which areas of your life you can gain clarity

You can gain clarity in any area of your life. It's totally up to you. We all have a few different areas of life where we need clarity. You know best in what areas of your life you need clarity the most. It can be obvious, but sometimes you may have to do a little digging. While finding your purpose is the main goal, gaining clarity in other areas of your life is essential to living more happy and setting yourself up for success.

You can go through all the areas of your life one by one. Pick one, get clear, and move on to the next. Going through different areas of your life where you need clarity will help you find your purpose. Here are some common areas and questions where you may need clarity:

Career

- How can I advance my career?
- Is it time for a promotion?
- Is this the right company for me?
- Should I change jobs?
- Should I go in a different direction with my career?
- Is there a possibility to work from home?
- Should I leave my job and stay at home with the kids?
- Should I start my own business? If so, what kind of business?
- Should I change jobs?

Relationships

- Do I want a relationship?
- Am I happy with my current relationship?

- How can I improve my relationship?

- Am I in love?

- Am I being treated fairly?

- Does this relationship drain my energy? Is it toxic?

- What about my friendships? Do they drain my energy? Am I surrounded by toxic people?

- Can this marriage be saved? Is it worth saving?

Family

- What are my family values?

- Do I want a partner?

- Do I want kids?

- Do I want to become married?

- How should I bring up my kids?

- Do I have a purpose other than being a parent?

Where to live?

- Where do I want to live?

- Where do I feel best?

- Should I be close to my family?

- Do I want to live alone or with someone?

- How much space do I need?

- What climate is best for me?

Finances

- How much money do I need to live comfortably? What does comfortable mean to me?

- What is financial freedom to me?

- How can I make money?

- Where is money on my priority list?

- How can I move forward and stop being stuck at my current income level?

Health

- Is my health in good condition?

- Do I feel healthy?

- Do I keep my weight in check? Am I overweight or underweight? If so, why?

- When do I feel my healthiest?

- Do I need help to improve my health?

How to find clarity

We always tend to follow the path that is most clear. However, it's not always the best choice. The right path is not always the one that is most obvious. Finding the right path requires asking yourself tough questions and listening to your intuition. You will have to ask yourself unusually specific questions in order to determine which path is the right one for you. Otherwise, you can end up going the path of least resistance, like most of us do - and no change will occur.

There are four elements to achieving clarity. Simply speaking, there has to be clarity about the who, the what, the why and the how.

The who?

The who is you obviously. You're the one looking for clarity. Of course, other people can be a part of your journey towards gaining clarity, but you are the main character. You will have to do all the work in order to gain clarity.

The what?

While it may seem rather simple, the what can be a complex subject. You can have a hundred different what's, from something simple like "I want to lose weight", to more complex questions like "What is my life mission?" Gaining total clarity requires you to answer the following questions:

- What is it that you really want?

- What is your purpose?

119

When you find answers to these questions, you will be able to establish your goals and tasks that you need to accomplish to achieve what you really want and fulfill your purpose.

The why?

While searching for your what's and trying to find your purpose, you have to figure out why. You probably won't be able to answer that question off the top of your head, and that's okay. Even if your what is something rather simple, like "I want to lose weight", you may think that your why is "because I want to look better" or "because I want to fit into my clothes". But it can go much deeper than that. Keep asking yourself why a few times and see how your answers gets simpler, yet deeper each time.

The how?

Once you've established what you want and why, now is the time to find a way how you can get there. You will have to create a plan, set goals and achieve them.

The process of finding clarity

You know what you need to gain clarity and now is the time to go through the whole process. It can be scary sometimes, but for the most part it's fun. We're actually closer to realizing what we want than we might think. But sometimes we are not ready to see it. Here are the practices that will help you gain clarity.

Self-reflection and awareness

In order to get clear about who you are and what you want, ask yourself the following questions and be completely honest with yourself:

- What do I feel unclear about?
- What do I need to help me get clear?

Next, listen to your body. See what it's trying to tell you about your physical, mental and emotional well-being? Do you always feel tired? Do you experience anxiety often? When? What triggers it?

Getting your thoughts on paper helps gain clarity. I personally find the brain dump method most effective. You can organize all things in your brain with a brain dump. Writing things down helps you set your priorities straight, clear your mind and organize your ideas.

A brain dump is essentially getting all your thoughts out of your head so that you can focus on one thing at a time. It helps you organize everything in your mind. Your tasks, your questions, your needs, your worries and everything that's important to you. These things can get stuck in your mind and distract you from what needs to be done. The aim of a brain dump is to establish everything you need and want to do. It's one of the ways to clear your mind, and it can be done in minutes. It will help you get organized and take control of your life.

If you keep all your thoughts in your head, your brain will keep going over them over and over again, making you feel overwhelmed in the process. It doesn't help if you want to achieve mental clarity. Take a brain dump, take all your scattered thoughts and get them all down, organize, and enjoy the clarity.

You can do a brain dump in five to ten minutes, so you can do it daily if you want to. Doing a brain dump at the end of the day is a great way to prepare yourself for the next day.

At the end of the day, take a look at what you've accomplished, what you've learned, and what you want to pursue tomorrow. Try doing a brain dump for five to ten minutes with no distractions or interruptions. If you can't do it daily, you can do a brain dump every few days or even weekly. You can do it at the end of each week, as it's the best time to note what you have accomplished and what you need to focus on next week.

You can also do a brain dump when you're starting to feel overwhelmed and need to get your thoughts down. Here are some examples when it's a good time to do a brain dump:

- When you're busy and need to prioritize tasks
- When you feel stuck
- When you feel overwhelmed
- When you're making plans in different areas of your life
- When you start learning something new
- When you find a big idea

Here's how you do a brain dump. It's a simple process. All you need is something you can write on: paper, whiteboard, or any electronic device you can type on.

First, start writing everything down. Dump your brain. Don't restrict yourself. Write down everything you need to do without any sort of priority. Write down your thoughts on what's going on. Write down what distracts you, what you fear, what is important to you. Write it all down.

After you're done writing it all down, take a small break for a minute. Now get back to your list and organizing everything. Organize it by grouping and prioritizing everything you've written down. You can group things into categories like work, family, friends, self-development, hobbies and so on.

And that's it. You've just done a brain dump. Keep practicing it and do it regularly, and it will become a habit. It can feel a bit overwhelming in the beginning, but you'll feel a sense of accomplishment after you've completed a brain dump. With time and practice, it will start feeling natural. Doing brain dumps regularly will help you move forward towards your goals and get things done.

Now, let's move on to the why and how you can dig deep to find it. Initially, asking yourself "why?", you will probably get a surface-level answer. To get to your true why, you simply have to keep asking. Here's an example. Let's say you want to lose weight. Why? Because I want to look better. Why? Because I want to feel better. Why? Because I want to feel self-conscious.

You have to keep going until you can't find any more answers and you think you've exhausted all of them. Your answers will keep getting more profound, meaningful and authentic. That is what clarity is all about.

And now we come to the how. Now that you have established what you want and why, it's time to set your goals and create a plan. Setting clear goals that will help you achieve your purpose is incredibly important. It's a topic I decided to dedicate a whole chapter to. We'll discuss how you can set your goals, develop strategies to achieve them, and maintain focus along the way in the next chapter. But first, let's finish talking about discovering your purpose with the help of clarity. Now that you know how to gain clarity in different areas of your life, it's time to think about your purpose.

Find your purpose

Finding your life purpose can be hard. There are a lot of problems in the world that need solving. There are a lot of people whom we could help support and inspire. There are a lot of passions you can pursue. Yet, finding your life purpose remains a difficult task.

There can be many reasons why you haven't discovered your life purpose yet. We've learned how you can discover yourself and gain clarity in order to find your purpose, yet it may still seem so distant. Maybe the world problems seem too big, or you think you're too small.

Maybe you feel exhausted from life and don't know where to find energy to pursue what really matters to you. However, finding your purpose and accomplishing it is the key to living a more happy, meaningful and fulfilling life.

Here are five steps you can take that will help you find your purpose:

1. Determine what drives you

When I was a student, I went to a bus stop after an exam and saw a student from my group sitting there. She was looking down into the ground and was squeezing her hand into a fist. I've noticed something dripping from her hand - it was blood!

So I rushed to her, grabbed her hand and opened it. It turned out she just grabbed a piece of broken glass from a bottle and she's been squeezing it as hard as she could. I realized she was intentionally trying to harm herself. She's always been quiet and rarely talked to anyone.

We went to get medical aid, and after a nurse mended her hand, we started talking. It turned out she's been so unhappy she just started harming herself. She tried her best and still didn't get a good enough grade in her opinion. Her parents were abusive, and she felt unhappy because she thought she was useless and couldn't achieve anything. She also revealed she attempted suicide multiple times but never told anyone. That was the moment that made me realize my purpose.

In the following years, I witnessed a lot more depression, mania and suicide attempts. I realized that a person can only take so much pain before becoming driven to stop it. Or at least that's what I thought.

Ask yourself the following question: What kind of pain, unhappiness or injustice have you witnessed that you can't live with? What touches you so deeply that it drives you? What can't you stand at all? Sometimes your purpose can come from painful experiences.

2. Discover what energizes you

It was a beautiful chilly morning. I woke up and started making a cup of coffee when I smelled a horrible stench of someone smoking a cigarette. Back then I used to live on the ground floor and the windows of my kitchen were right near the entrance to the building.

People often used to stand and smoke there. I hate the stench of cigarette smoke and it's illegal to smoke there. So I always had to ask people to move and smoke somewhere else. There was a big yard and most people were understanding. But not this time. When I asked them to leave and find another spot to smoke, they started cussing at me right away. They told to come out and handle it like a man, but at the same time they started walking away, cussing at me. I went to throw out the garbage a bit later and saw them standing behind a corner still cussing at me and giving me dirty looks.

The moral of the story is that you can burn your life if you pursue it in the wrong ways. Some ways deplete you rather than energize you. Instead of wasting your energy on unhelpful habits and behaviors, you should look for ways to energize yourself instead. With clarity, you may have found the problems you want to solve. Now it's time to think about how you can solve and where you can get energy to do it.

Ask yourself: what energizes you?

3. Think what you can sacrifice for

Have you ever thought about doing something, but never ending up following through or putting in the effort required to succeed? This does not necessarily have to be because of procrastination, laziness, or low self-confidence. We often neglect to do something because it's not important enough for us to sacrifice for.

For me, it happened when I decided to go to a graduate school to study psychiatry. I've seen a lot of pain and unhappiness caused by mental disorders in my life, and I wanted to learn how to solve them.

I studied hard to prepare for my graduate school applications, I studied even harder when I got into graduate school, I joined a research lab and I've been working hard every day until I passed out from exhaustion sometimes. I used to fall asleep at my desk studying. I had no personal life, no free time and no friends, and I don't regret it. I've found something I was willing to sacrifice for and it became my life purpose.

I must say I don't recommend you sacrificing to the point of burnout. You simply have to find something you're so passionate about that you're willing to sacrifice for it. Then you know you've found your purpose.

Ask yourself: what are you willing to sacrifice for?

4. Establish who you want to help

I've helped thousands of people in my life, and there is one thing I've noticed. I feel that I'm accomplishing my life purpose when I help change makers: people who will make the world a better place. I have a friend who was always eager to learn, always positive and excited to help others. I used to always support her when she studied, I helped her with her projects and I feel it was worth every second of my time. She's always striving to help others and make the world a better place. That's when I discovered that helping such people should be my priority, and now I focus on doing it.

Ask yourself: who do you want to help? Determining a person or a group of people you want to help will allow you to find your purpose more easily.

5. Determine how you want to help

I've worked with different people and companies and always used to do what I do best. But I've noticed it didn't energize me. However, with time I found my passion for content creation. I enjoy writing and creating. I can do it any time because I feel like it and it energizes me. I don't have to make myself do it.

So ask yourself: what is that you love doing? And how can you apply this passion to accomplish your purpose? You need to find out how you can use your skills, talents and passions to achieve your goals and accomplish your purpose.

Finding your purpose is a long but very exciting journey. It can take a lot of time and effort. So it's okay to take it one step at a time. It's okay to stop and reevaluate. It will not be easy, and you may encounter challenges along the way. You can even sometimes think of giving up and accepting defeat. But remember the first step. Think about what drives you and don't let yourself give up.

With that being said, let's move on to discussing how to set yourself up for success by setting clear goals that will allow you to develop your strategy and achieve your purpose.

Chapter 5: Set yourself up for success

How do you define success? Success is relative and can mean different things to different people. These days, we are being fed the information from the outside world on what society admires, praises and celebrates, yet we don't even think whether those accomplishments are what we truly aspire to achieve. We all can create and live fulfilling lives if we disregard what others think and reconnect with who we truly are.

You can use your strengths and preferences to your advantage and set yourself up for success, no matter how you define it. You can unleash your true potential when you discover your values and develop your strategy. All you have to do is take the first step today.

We've already discovered how you can discover yourself and find your purpose, and hopefully it will help you establish your true values, as it's the first step on the way to setting yourself up for success. You have to know what you want. Once you figure it out, you can find direction and the right path to take. And when you know where you're going, you can figure out how to get there.

You can set yourself up for success by devoting time and effort to what is most important to you. You just have to know how to achieve your goals and what tasks you have to accomplish along the way. Setting yourself up for success consists of four main steps. First, you need to discover your values. Then, you will learn how to set smart goals. Once you've done it, you'll discover how to develop your strategy to achieve those goals. And finally, you'll find out how you can stay focused along the way. These are the four elements of setting yourself up for success. Let's take a closer look at each of them.

Discover your values

Have you ever thought what your values and principles are? Before you can set clear goals, it's important to establish what's truly important to you. This will provide a clear framework for making decisions, because you can discard whatever isn't aligned with your values right from the start. It will help you exclude the unnecessary, narrow down your options and allow you to make decisions quicker and more effectively. Consider your values taking your passions into account. This way you can stay true to your values, while following your passions and fulfilling your life purpose. Discovering your values is important for the following reasons:

- You will feel more ownership over what you're doing
- You will gain more motivation and better focus
- You will have greater dedication and commitment
- You will have a positive outlook and expectation
- You will find more pleasure doing what you truly enjoy

Our values are a part of us. They are the highlight of what we stand for. They represent your unique character, preferences, and your essence. Our behavior is guided by our values. You can live a more happy and fulfilling life when you honor your personal values. When we don't, we are more likely to indulge in bad habits and unhelpful destructive behavior.

I started discovering my values when I first noticed my health started deteriorating. I've gained a lot of weight during my studies at the university and my vision got pretty bad from all the reading, writing and sitting in front of a computer all day. I attended a seminar on values one day, and that was when I discovered I need to make my health my priority. It's the value that I put on top of my list that day.

I committed to eating a healthy diet and started exercising. I also started caring about my vision by having regular breaks and not sitting for hours reading or staring into a computer screen. Although my vision isn't perfect and it will probably never be without laser eye surgery, it still improved noticeably, and my eyes no longer hurt after a long day at work. Apart from that, I decided to create a foundation to maintain my health by introducing healthy habits, such as taking regular breaks, going for a walk in the morning and having enough sleep.

Establishing this value as my top priority changed my life. It changed my diet and my habits. I feel so much better now, and I know I can maintain my health in good condition for years to come if I maintain it as one of my top priorities.

These days people value comfort. Our society is ingrained with the idea that the more we have and the more comfortable our lives are, the more happy we are. But growth does not come from comfort. When people choose comfort over growth, they become stuck and unwilling to grow and change. Now think what can happen when people choose comfort over health. Eating to feel better and indulging in destructive habits will destroy one's health. That's why it's important to determine your values first. This way, you will be able to set clear goals and develop your strategy to succeed.

Discover your core values

These days most of us don't know our values. We don't know what's truly important to us. As a result, we can accept the values instilled by our culture, society and media. Can you name your values off the top of your head? In my experience, it's a difficult task for most people.

It's hard to determine your values without going through a discovery process. You can speculate and idealize what you should value, but discovering your true core values takes time and effort.

You can do it if you're ready to be completely honest with yourself and if you have patience and determination. You can write down your thoughts or take notes if you find it useful during the whole process. I suggest doing so. Take something you can write or type on and let's get started. Here are seven steps you should take to discover your true core values.

1. Start with a beginner's mind

We tend to presume that we know the answers to many questions, but in reality, that's usually not the case. Before you embark on a personal and creative journey to discover your values, you have to adopt a beginner's mindset. You have to dismiss all your preconceived notions in order to gain access to your inner truths.

Take a deep breath and clear your mind. Remember that your conscious mind doesn't have all the answers. You have to clear your mind in order to make space for new insights. Getting into the right mental state is an important first step.

2. Create a list of your personal values

Making a short and concise list of personal values can be a difficult task. If you look online, you can find lists with hundreds of values. But I don't recommend going through any predetermined lists. After all, you don't select values - you discover them. If you go through a predetermined list of values, your brain will evaluate them and make it seem like some are better than others.

However, if you're totally lost or not familiar with values, you can go through a list to get a sense of what you might be looking for. Here are three techniques you can try to discover your own personal values:

Peak experiences

Think of your peak experiences - meaningful moments that stand out. What was happening? What was going on? By which values were you guided at that time?

Suppressed values

Now think of the opposite - remember when you were angry, frustrated or upset. What was happening then? What were you feeling? What value was being suppressed?

Code of conduct

Think about what's most important to you beyond basic human needs. What do you need to experience fulfillment? It can be a lot of things. Creative self-expression, strong health, a sense of adventure, aspiration to learn and discover or create beauty.

3. Gather your personal values into related groups

Now that you've made a list of your personal values, it's time to gather your values into related groups. First, see how many values are on your list. There can be dozens of values, but that's too many to be actionable. Five to ten personal values seems to be the magic number.

We will discuss how to determine your most important values a bit later, but now let's gather them into related groups. For instance, values like responsibility and accountability are related. Values like learning, growth and development are related too. Gather your values into related groups.

4. Determine the main theme of each group

Think what word or words best represent each group of your values. For example, if you have values like learning, growth and development, self-development is the main theme of these values. Go through each of the groups and name them.

5. Establish your top personal values

You may have quite a long list of values. Here are a few questions that can help narrow your list of values down:

- What values are essential to you?

- What values represent your way of being?

- What values are essential to supporting your inner self?

I suppose you might be wondering how many values you should have at this point. If there are too few, you will not capture all your unique preferences. If there are too many, it's usually not actionable and you will neglect some of them. While there is no specific number of values you should have, the magic number seems to be from five to ten. It's usually enough to represent what you stand for and be actionable at the same time.

Now comes the most difficult part. You have to rank your values in the order of importance. You don't have to do it all at once. Do one round and then put your list aside. Come back to it later and go through the process again.

6. Give your values broader context

Now you'll have to be creative. Turning your values into memorable phrases or slogans can help you establish the meaning behind each value. You can make it more memorable and personal this way. Here's how you can make your values statements:

- Use inspiring words and phrases - our brains are naturally attracted to something that looks and sounds powerful and unique, rather than something mundane.

- Find words that trigger emotional responses, as they will be more memorable and meaningful.

- Make your statements inspire you, make them rich and meaningful.

- Play around your strengths when making statements.

For instance, if one of your core values is health, well-being and vitality, your statement could look like this: "Health: living with full vitality and takeing care of my well-being every day".

7. Take a step back and examine each of your values

After you've completed your list of your top core values, set it aside and examine it the next day after a good night's sleep. Ask yourself the following questions:

- How do they make you feel?
- Are these values consistent with who you are?
- Are they personal to you?
- Are there any values that are inconsistent with your identity, as if they belong to someone else, like an authority figure or society, and not you?
- Check the priority ranking, are your values in the correct order of importance?

Make any changes if necessary. Knowing your core values will help you make decisions in all areas of your life.

Set your goals

Now that you know your values and passions, it's time to set specific goals that will help you get where you want to be. Have you ever thought what your goals are? Where do you see yourself in five years? Do you know what your main objective is?

You need to set goals if you want to succeed. Without goals, you will lack direction and focus. They also provide you with milestones and benchmarks to determine whether you've actually succeeded. Success is relative and has a different meaning to different people. If your goal is to accumulate riches, then having a million dollars is the proof of your success. But if your goal is doing charitable acts, then keeping money for yourself contradicts your goal.

You need to know how to set your goals before you can accomplish them. You can't simply say "I want it" and expect it to happen. Setting goals starts with determining what you want to achieve and ends with a lot of effort and hard work to get there. Here are five steps to setting specific goals that will help you build your way to success:

1. Set goals to motivate yourself

It's important to set goals what will motivate you. They have to be important to you, and there should be value in achieving them. If you have little interest in achieving some goals, they can become irrelevant, and it's highly likely you will not put in the effort required to achieve them. Motivation is an important part to achieving goals.

Set goals that are aligned with your values, priorities, and passions. You have to commit to reaching your goals, and when they are in line with what's truly important to you, it gives you a sense of urgency and maximizes your chances to succeed. When you don't have this, you'll have a tendency of putting off taking action to achieve your goals. This is turn will make you frustrated and disappointed. Make sure to set motivating goals in order to maximize your chances to succeed.

2. Set SMART goals

It's possible you've heard about SMART goals. But even if you have, do you follow this rule? Have you ever tried applying it at all? SMART stands for:

- Specific
- Measurable
- Attainable
- Relevant

- Time Bound

Set specific goals

Your goals must be clear and specific because they provide direction. Your goals need to show you the way. That's why setting vague or generalized goals is unhelpful, as they don't provide direction. Setting specific goals will make it easy for you to get where you want to go because they precisely define where you want to end up.

Set measurable goals

Setting measurable goals allows you to measure the degree of your success. If you have a goal to improve your income, how will you know when you have succeeded? Even a 1% increase in your earnings is technically a success. You need to set specific measurable goals whenever possible so that you have a way to measure the degree of your success. Going back to increasing your income goal, it should look like this: increase my income by 10% in a year. This is a specific measurable goal, and you can measure your success and know whether you have actually achieved what you wanted.

Set attainable goals

Setting attainable goals means you should make sure you set goals that are possible to achieve. If you set goals that you can't achieve, you will only destroy your self-confidence and demoralize yourself.

On the other hand, you shouldn't be looking to set goals that are too easy. Reaching goals that don't require a lot of effort to achieve is anticlimactic at best, and it can make you afraid of setting more challenging goals in the future. You need to find a balance by setting challenging but realistic goals. In order to achieve such goals, you will have to become more than you were before and raise the bar. Achieving these goals brings the greatest satisfaction and makes you improve constantly.

Set relevant goals

Your goals should be relevant to the direction you want your life to take. If you keep your goals aligned with your values, priorities and passions, you'll be able to develop the focus and consistency to get ahead and do what needs to be done. If you set inconsistent and widely scattered goals, you'll waste your time and effort pursuing something you don't really need or have little use for.

Set time-bound goals

Similarly to how your goals should be measurable, they also should have a deadline or timeframe within which they should be achieved. Once again, it will allow you to measure the degree of success. In addition to that, working on a deadline gives you a sense of urgency and provides motivation, which will keep you focused and more consistent.

3. Write down your goals

Writing down your goals will help make them real and tangible. If they are written right here in front of you, you will not have any excuses for forgetting about them. When writing down your goals, use the word "will", and not "would like to", or "need to". For instance, I will reduce my expenses by 10% this year. Goals formulated in this manner have power, and you can literally see yourself reducing the expenses.

If you use a to-do list, make a template that has your goals at the top. You can also place reminders in visible places to remind yourself every day of what you need to do. Put them at your desk, near your computer screen, on your walls, on your refrigerator or on your bathroom mirror as a constant reminder.

4. Make an action plan

This step is crucial, but it's often missed when setting goals. You get so concentrated on the result that you forget to plan all the steps that are required to actually achieve the desired result. You should create an action plan by writing down individual steps. It will provide additional motivation, as you will be crossing out each step after completing it and seeing your progress towards your ultimate goal. This is especially important if your goal is big and demanding, or long-term.

Start by determining all the tasks that need to be completed to achieve your goal. Think what's the first action you have to take. Once it's done, what comes next? Are there any steps that need to be prioritized to meet specific deadlines? You should end up with a list of tasks that you need to complete to reach your goal, in the order that you need to complete them.

5. Review your goals and action plans from time to time to make sure they remain relevant

Remember that setting goals is only the beginning. Create reminders to keep yourself on track and review your goals regularly. Setting goals is an ongoing activity, and even though your goal may remain the same in the long-term, the action plan can change.

Setting goals is much more than simply saying you want something to happen. You have to define exactly what you want and why you want it in order to maximize your chances of succeeding. By following these five rules, you'll be able to set smart goals that will motivate you and enjoy the confidence and satisfaction you get from achieving those goals.

\#

Develop your strategy

Now that you know how to set smart goals, let's take a look at how you can develop your strategy to reach those goals. You will have to assess your current situation. First, it's important to consider how different goals relate to each other. Make sure that your professional and financial goals don't take away from family, relationship or spiritual goals in your life. It's important to find a balance between different areas of your life. You will also have to consider what assets you currently have and what you need to obtain to achieve your goals. Also, consider what obstacles you may have to face along the way and don't allow them to become excuses for not reaching your goals.

Here are nine ways that will help you develop your strategy and follow through. While some of them may seem fairly simple and straightforward, others require more effort.

1. Create a plan

We've discussed how planning is an essential step in goal setting. Your chances of achieving anything without planning are close to zero. Achieving your goals requires ample planning, so that you know what direction you're heading and how you can get where you need to be. However, you don't necessarily need to know every step you have to take.

Let's take flights and airplanes, for example. Planes need to take off and land in a specific city, on a specific date and at a specific time. In order to achieve that goal, planes need to make a plan - a flight plan. But the flight plan can change. It only accounts for some variables, such as fuel consumption, flight speed, altitude and travel course. But things can change along the way due to air turbulence, traffic congestion, and other factors. So the flight plan needs to be adjusted accordingly.

In a similar manner, you'll have to create a plan in order to reach your goals, but remember it can and most likely will need to be adjusted along the way. You don't have to change your goals, unless they become irrelevant at some point due to various circumstances. But you can and you should change your plan in accordance with the current conditions and circumstances in order to make progress towards your goals.

2. Discipline

Achieving goals without proper discipline is nearly impossible. Even if you set your goals the right way, without disciple, it's highly likely you will not follow through. You can improve your discipline by introducing the right habits into your life.

You need order and organization in order to achieve discipline. When things are disorganized, it becomes much harder to maintain focus and stay on track. Order and organization create discipline, which in turn helps you reach your goals.

This is easier said than done, of course. However, we've discussed how you can simplify your life and gain clarity in order to defeat disorganization. Improving your discipline and organization is not an overnight process. You can always go back to the previous chapters to review the tips on how to improve your discipline and organization.

3. Eliminate distractions

It's easy to get distracted, especially in the modern world. Different things can pull us in different directions.

We can get pulled off course and veer from one thing after another. It's obvious that distractions hurt your chances of achieving your goals. You need to lessen the distractions in your life in order to remain focused.

Determine where distractions are coming from in your life, and work on eliminating the ones that take up most of your valuable time. Some common examples are aimlessly scrolling through social media, channel surfing, binge-watching movies or TV series, excessive socializing and other time-wasting activities.

Removing the distractions will allow you to find more valuable time to pursue your goals instead of wasting it at things that don't really matter. It doesn't mean you should always work without rest, that's unhealthy. You should take regular breaks, have a good rest and sleep well. But try doing useful things during your breaks, like exercising a little or going for a walk rather than wasting your time aimlessly staring into your phone, for example. You probably know how much of your free time is being wasted already and what distractions are causing this. Do your best to eliminate them.

4. Set milestones

Milestones are helpful signposts that you should set on the way to your goals. You can take some long-term goals and break it up into milestones. You can create weekly or monthly milestones and other benchmarks that are relevant to your goals.

It's much easier to create milestones if you have measurable goals. You can break up your goals into equal parts. For instance, if you want to lose 30 pounds in 6 months, you need to lose 5 pounds a month. Your weight loss may not be linear like that, but now you have a benchmark that will allow you to stay on track and measure the degree of your success.

Milestones are also helpful because they allow you to see short-term results on the way to long-term goals. They make your progress measurable and manageable, as long-term goals can sometimes seem too big and overwhelm you. Milestones allow you to actually gauge your progress on the way to success.

5. Overcome procrastination

All of us are familiar with the feeling of procrastination. Procrastination is the silent killer of goal achievement. If you let procrastination overwhelm you, the chances of you achieving your goals become zero.

Procrastination is a natural tendency of putting things off, but it doesn't mean you should allow it to overwhelm you. You have to do what it takes to get rid of procrastination.

It's obvious you won't reach any goals by procrastinating. If you have a tendency to put things off until the last minute, try implement the 15-minute rule. Remove any distractions, set a timer for 15 minutes and dedicate this time to doing something that needs to be done.

This way you can develop a useful habit and build momentum. You start with a small commitment, but it makes you move in the direction you need to go. In many cases, you will find that after those 15 minutes you'll keep going. Once you occupy yourself with something, it's highly likely you will keep going until it's done. An object in motion tends to stay in motion. Give it a try today.

6. Manage your time effectively

Time management is important to achieve your goals. If you implement this strategy well enough, it will help you reach even the most ambitious goals. There many good systems for managing your time, but the one I personally found works well is the Pomodoro technique.

It is a sort of extension of the 15-minute rule to overcome procrastination. It helps you avoid distractions and interruptions, which is one of the reasons why people are unable to maximize their productivity. With this technique, you focus on your work in short bursts of time. The idea is to put your tasks into 25-minute intervals of uninterrupted work with 5-minute breaks in between. Having a timer in front of you helps you become more focused on getting the job done and even beating the clock.

Here's how it works. Get a timer and set it to 25 minutes, work uninterrupted during this period, and then take a 5-minute bread afterwards. For this to work you have to keep working even if you're tempted to extend the interval or even quit. You also need to take regular 5-minute breaks after 25 minuted of work. This time management technique helps you avoid distractions and utilize your valuable time effectively.

You can consider other techniques, of course. There are many time management techniques, such as time blocking, Getting Things Done, bullet journal, and so on. You have to find a technique or a combination of techniques that work best for you.

7. Complete most important tasks in the morning

Your most important tasks are the things you can do to advance towards achieving your long-term goals now. In time management, they are important but not urgent tasks. If you have such tasks, it's best to do them first thing in the morning. If you have multiple important tasks, you should tackle the biggest or most difficult first. Focus on completing your most important tasks in the mornings and you'll progress towards achieving your goals steadily and quickly.

8. Implement the 80/20 rule

According to the 80/20 rule, also known as the Pareto Principle, 80% of the results come from 20% of the effort. In sales, this also means that 80% of the sales come from 20% of the clients. You have to identify this 20% of your efforts that will produce 80% of your results and focus on them.

To identify them, you will have to take a close look at your activities related to your goals. See what efforts you are putting in and what results your getting from them. To determine this properly, you will have to constantly measure your results. This is not a simple procedure, but when you identify the efforts you should focus on, you will take your results to the next level.

9. Anticipate failure

Failure is common when trying to achieve goals, and that's fine. Failure is a wise teacher, and you should learn from it. It's often difficult to deal with failure, because we usually don't anticipate it. However, if you can anticipate failure, you will be able to deal with it more effectively and adjust your plans accordingly.

The most successful people have failed the most times. Failure is a part of your way to success, and it should be anticipated. This way, you will be able to use it as stepping stones, instead of dwelling on it wasting your time and energy.

Most importantly, be consistent and don't give up. You can overcome your failures and stay focused on your goals. With persistency and determination, you will reach your goals.

Stay focused

All successful people have one trait in common - focus. Focus is a skill that allows you to take charge of your life despite any setbacks, distractions or fears, and remain set on achieving your goals. Focus is what helps you concentrate on your goals and doing what's necessary to achieve them. If you're focused, you will pursue your goals with passion and appreciate your progress on the way to achieving them. Being focused doesn't mean focusing solely on your goals and neglecting other areas of your life, though. It means focusing on the right things and not getting distracted by unhelpful or irrelevant issues and ideas. Here are some examples:

- Instead of focusing on your ego or personal status, focus on doing the job right

- Instead of focusing on your past mistakes or future worries, focus on what is required now and what you can do now

- Instead of focusing on being perfect, focus on being exceptional and doing your best

- Instead of focusing on why something didn't go right, focus on how you can fix the problem

- Instead of focusing on what you can't do well, focus on your self-worth and strengths

Regardless of what success means to you, it is important to learn how to take control of your life and make change when required. When you're truly passionate about something and you are willing to put in the effort - you know you are on the right track. You have a great plan, you've developed a strategy on how you're planning to reach your goals, all you have to do now is stay focused and stick with it even through difficult times. Remember why you've decided to set your goals in the first place and don't allow anyone to take you off course.

Why focus is important

Having focus is important because distraction and switching leads to your time being wasted. The day goes by, but you've barely accomplished anything important. Spending days procrastinating and getting pulled off by distractions is the worst that can happen. Your time is the most valuable resource you have and your life is too precious to waste, so you want to stay focused on what's truly important to you.

Staying focused on a single task at a time will help you get things done. We are naturally pulled towards procrastination and important tasks tend to get pushed back. Staying focused on your tasks will improve your personal effectiveness and will allow you to progress towards achieving your goals at a quick pace.

If you tend to procrastinate, if you feel stressed out by all the tasks you have to do, then improving your focus will help you in a big way. Let's move on to how you can actually stay focused.

Many things are required in orders to succeed, but willpower and determination are the most important. People think that we are born with determination and successful people were simply fortunate to be born with an abundant supply of determination. That is not true. Some people are not born with more determination than others, they simply find a way to harness and use what they have more effectively. Here are five ways that will help you harness your determination and improve your focus.

1. Get prepared for the day ahead the night before

Before going to sleep, plan what you will do the next day. Decide what you will wear, what you will eat, and how you will get where you need to go. It's much easier if you get your clothes prepared the night before and pack a healthy lunch instead of going for a takeout. The same principle applies when spending money. Create a budget and stick to it.

Make a decision the night before that you will do your most important tasks first and everything else later. Stick to your schedule and avoid distractions. Planning your day ahead will make you more organized and you will gain more time to complete the important tasks, instead of getting sidetracked and wasting your time and energy on unimportant things.

2. Do the most difficult tasks first

Difficult tasks will not get any easier the longer you put them off. You will only waste time and energy that would be better spent tackling the task head on. Do your most difficult tasks first while you're fresh and full of energy.

Research shows that our minds perform best in the morning, and that is the best time for tackling the hardest tasks. Once you've completed them, you can move on to more routine work that doesn't require that much effort. After that, don't forget to relax and practice some self-care.

3. Avoid distractions

Real emergencies can come up and you will have to deal with them. However, most situations that do come up are not emergencies and you don't have to respond right away. Sometimes they may even resolve themselves on their own with time.

Responding to such requests right away will only set you up to receive more. By not responding, you're sending a message that you are very busy and over time you should get bothered less by trivial matters.

4. Remember to rest and keep up your energy

Remember to take regular breaks when working on something. Take a break if you feel your energy fading. If you need to clear your mind, take a walk or do some exercise to take a brief retreat from work and regenerate. You will get back to work energized and with a sharper focus.

Instead of eating a large meal at lunch, try eating smaller portions and snack on healthy foods throughout the day. Eating a large meal can make you feel tired and sleepy, as your body will have to spend a lot of energy on digesting all the food you've consumed. As a result, you'll feel groggy and it will be much harder to maintain focus and concentrate of your tasks. Remember to hydrate yourself, drink water whenever you feel thirsty. With time, you'll develop healthy habits that will allow you to keep up your energy and maintain sharp focus throughout the day.

5. Remind yourself of your ultimate goals

Create reminders in visible places to keep yourself motivated and constantly remind yourself what you are working toward. You can also include your "why" behind the goal.

Let's say you want to increase your earnings by 10% in a year. Have a clear vision of how you will do that. Will you get a promotion or start a side gig? Remember why you want that. What will you do with the extra income? Will you invest it or is there something you need to purchase? Spend a couple of minutes daily visualizing your goals. Imagine it in as much detail as possible. It's a great technique to motivate yourself and keep moving forward toward your goals.

The lack of focus can really put a dent in your productivity. That's why it's important to know a few simple yet effective techniques to stay focused. Knowing how to focus on what needs to be done will help you stay on track and reach your goals.

Conclusion

In conclusion, let's summarize all the valuable strategies and techniques we've discovered that can help you live more happy, discover yourself, simplify your life and focus on what matters to you.

The first step on the way to living a more happy and fulfilling life is discovering yourself. Discovering your identity, discovering who you really are, is the greatest and most important adventure of your life. However, many of us don't realize that and walk around not really knowing who we truly are. In order to become the best version of yourself and succeed in various aspects of life, you first have to know who you really are, what your values are, and what you have to offer to the people surrounding you and the world. When you discover yourself, you will discover your true values and goals. You will know what you need to do in order to achieve them. Discovering yourself allows you to avoid lots of frustration caused by putting time and effort into the wrong things. Once you discover yourself, you will gain more confidence in your abilities and will begin setting yourself up for success.

Discovering yourself involves a lot of self-reflection. You will have to make time for solitude, make sense of your past, and purge yourself mentally and emotionally. There are various techniques that can help you discover yourself, such as embracing your right to be self-sovereign, determining what you really want in life and asking yourself self-discovery questions. Discovering yourself can be a difficult journey, but it's surely an incredibly fascinating one, and everyone will benefit from taking it. You'll find out who you truly are, what you stand for, what your values are, and what you true needs and goals are. Self-discovery is a fascinating journey, and it is the first step on the way to living more happy and focusing on what truly matters to you.

Next, it's essential to make yourself your top priority and dismiss the mistaken belief that self-care is selfish. We often fail to notice, but most people are actually better at taking care of other people than taking care of ourselves. Most of us are bad at prioritizing our own needs over the needs of people around us. But think, where does it leave you? The answer is tired, stressed and frustrated. Because you didn't leave enough time for you in all your attempts to help everyone else. This is why you should make yourself your number one priority. This is why you must become the most important person in your life. You have to take care of yourself before you can help everyone else. You can't perform at your best if you're tired, stressed, and frustrated.

There are a few different ways to prioritize yourself. First, you have to realize that self-care is essential to your well-being and is not selfish. Then you can start making non-negotiable rules, such as making morning your "me" time. Before you go anywhere or do anything, take care of yourself first. Have a nice breakfast, go for a walk or do some exercise, or simply look out of the window with a cup of hot tea and do some self-reflection. Do not over-schedule yourself, do what's important to you first, and discard the rest. Find some time to be alone sometimes. It's nice to take a break once in a while and take some time for yourself to explore your feelings and grow personally. Set boundaries and learn to say no. Remember, self-care doesn't have to look a certain way. You can find different ways to take care of your needs that suit you best. The most important thing is that you make it a habit. Always remember that you matter, your life matters, your needs and desires matter. When you take care of yourself, you are in a much better position to help others.

Now that you know how to prioritize yourself, it's time to move on to simplifying your life, so that you can make more space and focus on the things that matter to you and discard the rest. Simplifying your life is important because everything in your life takes space, time and energy. Everything you do, everything you own and everyone you spend time with costs you something - time, energy, money. And when you have a lot of stuff, it costs you a lot. These days, our society reinforces the idea that the more we own, the happier we will become. In reality, most of us have more than we really need. Simplifying your life will allow you to find more time, space and energy.

There are many ways you can simplify your life, and just like self-care, simplifying your life doesn't have to look a certain way. You can choose what works best in your circumstances. You can start by decluttering your house and getting rid of the things that you don't use or are broken. You can remove toxic people from your life. If someone is draining your energy and only adds negativity to your life, you need to evaluate whether you want to spend time with them at all. In addition to removing unnecessary things and toxic people from your life, you can also consider reducing the number of commitments. If you're struggling with running a carpool or having too many meetings, learn to say no. It's great to give back and spend time with your friends, but it's also important to have healthy boundaries, so that you can focus on the thing that are truly important to you. You can eliminate bad mental habits, such as negative self-talk and stop wasting time on being negative, as it doesn't help and you should learn from your mistakes and not dwell on them. Start removing one thing from your life every day. Get rid of some clutter, cut out toxic people, spend some time alone and clear your mind.

Now that you know how you can simplify your life to create more time and space for what's important to you, it's time to move on to learning how to gain clarity. We often find ourselves confused in the fast-paced, frantic modern world. Gaining clarity will help you discover your purpose and your passions, and find out what exactly is important to you and how you can achieve it. Finding your purpose is one of the greatest feelings in life. It starts with gaining clarity about who you are and what you want. Once you've established that, you can set goals that will allow you to pursue your purpose. Unfortunately, with the hectic modern lifestyle, most of us don't even think about who we are and what our purpose is. You can gain clarity by answering four questions: Who? What? Why? and How? Who is you, because you are the one who wants to gain clarity. What is what you want and what your purpose is. Why is why you want it. And how is how you're going to achieve what you want. Finding your purpose can be a long journey, but it's a very exciting one. With that being said, it's time to move on to setting yourself up for success by setting clear goals that will allow you to develop your strategy and achieve your purpose.

Success is relative and can mean different things to different people. No matter how you define success, there are simple actions you can take to build on your natural preferences and strengths, guided by your true values and desires, and created by you in a way that would set you up for success. You can set yourself up for success by discovering your values, setting clear goals, and developing your strategy on how to achieve them and staying focus along the way. Before you can set clear goals, it's important to establish what's truly important to you - your values. This will provide a clear framework for making decisions, because you can discard whatever isn't aligned with your values right from the start. It will help you exclude the unnecessary, narrow down your options and allow you to make decisions quicker and more effectively.

Now that you know your values and passions, it's time to set specific goals and help you get where you want to be. You need to set goals if you want to succeed. Without goals, you will lack direction and focus. They also provide you with milestones and benchmarks to determine whether you've actually succeeded. You should set specific, measurable, attainable, relevant and time-bound goals. Once you've set clear goals, it's time to develop the strategy of how to reach them. First, it's important to consider how different goals relate to each other. Make sure that your professional and financial goals don't take away from family, relationship or spiritual goals in your life. It's important to find a balance between different areas of your life. You will also have to consider what assets you currently have and what you need to obtain to achieve your goals. Also, consider what obstacles you may have to face along the way and don't allow them to become excuses for not reaching your goals. And finally, you'll have to learn how to stay focused in order to achieve your goals. Focus is a skill that allows you to take charge of your life despite and setbacks, distractions or fears, and remain set on achieving your goals. Focus is what helps you concentrate on your goals and doing what's necessary to achieve them. You have a great plan, you've developed a strategy on how you're planning to reach your goals, all you have to do now is stay focused and stick with it even through difficult times. Remember why you've decided to set your goals in the first place and don't allow anyone to take you off course.

18866776R00095